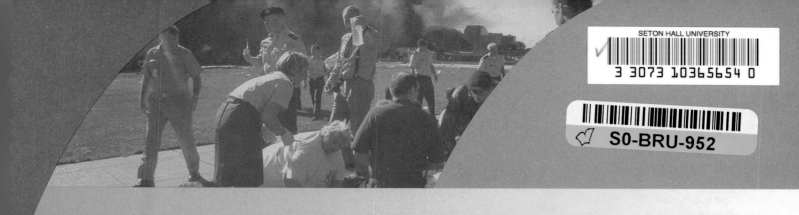

Essentials of Public Health Preparedness

Rebecca Katz, MPH, PhD

Assistant Professor
George Washington University
School of Public Health and Health Services
Washington, DC

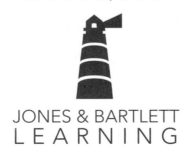

JONES & BARTLETT
LEARNING

World Headquarters
Jones & Bartlett Learning
5 Wall Street
Burlington, MA 01803
978-443-5000
info@jblearning.com
www.jblearning.com

Jones & Bartlett Learning books and products are available through most bookstores and online booksellers. To contact Jones & Bartlett Learning directly, call 800-832-0034, fax 978-443-8000, or visit our website, www.jblearning.com.

Substantial discounts on bulk quantities of Jones & Bartlett Learning publications are available to corporations, professional associations, and other qualified organizations. For details and specific discount information, contact the special sales department at Jones & Bartlett Learning via the above contact information or send an email to specialsales@jblearning.com.

This publication is designed to provide accurate and authoritative information in regard to the Subject Matter covered. It is sold with the understanding that the publisher is not engaged in rendering legal, accounting, or other professional service. If legal advice or other expert assistance is required, the service of a competent professional person should be sought.

Production Credits
Publisher: Michael Brown
Managing Editor: Maro Gartside
Editorial Assistant: Chloe Falivene
Production Manager: Tracey McCrea
Associate Marketing Manager: Jody Sullivan
Manufacturing and Inventory Control Supervisor: Amy Bacus
Composition: Publishers' Design and Production Services, Inc.

Cover Design: Kristin E. Parker
Rights & Photo Research Manager: Katherine Crighton
Photo Research Supervisor: Anna Genoese
Cover Image: © Caitlin Mirra/ShutterStock, Inc.
Section and Chapter Opener Image: Courtesy of Journalist 1st Class Mark D. Faram/U.S. Navy
Printing and Binding: Malloy, Inc.
Cover Printing: Malloy, Inc.

Library of Congress Cataloging-in-Publication Data
Katz, Rebecca Lynn, 1973–
    Essentials of public health preparedness / Rebecca Katz.
        p. ; cm.
    Includes bibliographical references and index.
    ISBN-13: 978-0-7637-7983-2 (pbk.)
    ISBN-10: 0-7637-7983-0 (pbk.)
  1. Public health—United States. 2. Disaster medicine—United States. 3. Public health administration—United States. 4. Civil defense readiness—United States. I. Title.
    [DNLM: 1. Civil Defense—United States. 2. Disaster Planning—United States. 3. Public Health Administration—United States. 4. Security Measures—United States. 5. Terrorism—prevention & control—United States. WA 295]
    RA445.K34 2012
    363.34'8—dc23
        2011014807
6048
Printed in the United States of America
15   14   13   12   11   10 9 8 7 6 5 4 3 2 1

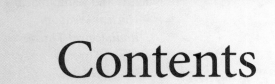

Contents

Prologue: *Essentials of Public Health Preparedness*

Public Health is no longer exclusively about promoting health and preventing disease; it is now about protecting health as well. From bioterrorism to environmental disasters and emerging communicable disease, threats to health now appear everywhere we look. *Essentials of Public Health Preparedness* takes an all-hazards approach to public health preparedness, providing broad perspectives on local, national, and global threats.

Professor Katz takes on the challenge of putting public health preparedness in the larger context of public health education and public policy. She brings to this challenge a wealth of background in the policy aspects of public health preparedness, having worked at the intersection of infectious diseases and national security for the Defense Intelligence Agency, the Joint Military Intelligence College, and the Department of State. Rebecca Katz builds on an exceptional education background at Swarthmore (BA), Yale (MPH), and Princeton (PhD).

Essentials of Public Health Preparedness focuses on public policy but does not stop there. Dr. Katz goes on to describe the operational aspects of public health preparedness. She reviews the experience of September 11, 2001 and the recommendations of the 9/11 Commission, exploring the framework and institutions being built on these recommendations. Once the reader has understood the basics, she turns her attention to solving problems. In doing this she develops in the reader an appreciation of the complexities of the issues that must be considered by public health professionals in designing preparedness and response plans, policies, regulations, and legislation.

The text concludes with a look at what can be learned from recent experiences. Pandemic influenza and Hurricane Katrina represent two episodes that help illustrate the wide range of interventions and policies that are needed to protect health. They also illustrate the essential roles that the public health community plays in preparing for and responding to security threats.

Essentials of Public Health Preparedness assumes no prior background in public health preparedness, yet it speaks to the needs of undergraduate students, graduate students, and public health practitioners. Public health preparedness has become a cornerstone of public health and a major undertaking of governmental public health. Public health preparedness content is increasingly being integrated into public health education at the undergraduate, as well as graduate levels. New competencies are been developed by the Association of School of Public Health with support and encouragement from Centers for Disease Control and Prevention. *Essentials of Public Health Preparedness* will help students and practitioners fulfill these competencies.

I'm confident that you will find this book engaging and enlightening. I'm delighted that *Essentials of Public Health Preparedness* is now a part of our Essential Public Health series.

Richard Riegelman, MD, MPH, PhD
Series Editor, *Essential Public Health*

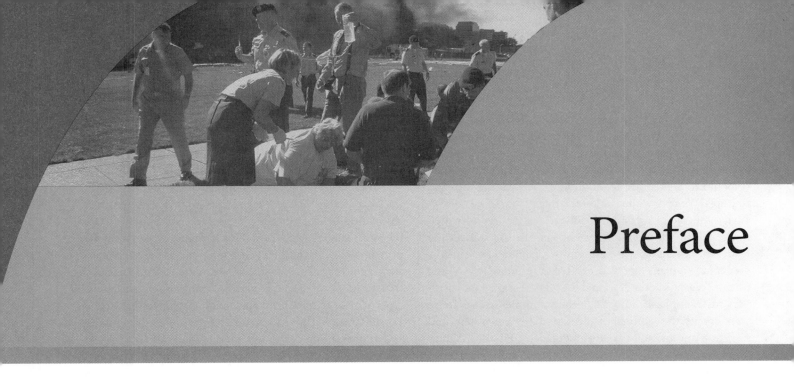

Preface

The last decade has seen many changes in terms of how we view our security and the role of the public health community. There is an ever-evolving threat of the terrorist use of weapons of mass destruction against our population, in particular the use of biological weapons. Infectious diseases continue to emerge and reemerge around the world, and the globalization of our food supply and the speed and volume of international travel make us all vulnerable to the emergence of a new agent anywhere in the world.

There is mounting evidence that large-scale epidemics can dramatically affect the economic, social, and security foundations of a nation. We are constantly reminded of the devastating effects of natural disasters, particularly hurricanes and earthquakes. All of these factors have led to the emergence of a new subdiscipline within public health—public health preparedness. The public health community plays a vital role in identifying, responding to, containing, and recovering from emergencies. It is imperative that public health professionals develop an awareness of the emerging threats, the means of addressing those threats, and the security challenges inherent in these activities and that they be able to identify and work with other sectors with similar responsibilities.

Public health preparedness is a new discipline, but it has been rapidly developing at the federal, state, and local levels. Academia is now acknowledging this as an essential area of expertise necessary for a fully developed public health workforce. The goal of this book is to introduce students to the field of public health preparedness. The book presupposes no previous exposure to the concepts, yet provides enough depth for students who may have advanced knowledge.

Public Health Preparedness is divided into four parts:

Part I: Background of the Field
Part II: Defining the Problem: Potential Threats
Part III: Infrastructure
Part IV: Solving Problems

Part I provides an overview and background to the field of public health preparedness. We look at how the field has evolved, as well as how different entities have defined the subdiscipline. We also review the definitions and evolution of national security and homeland security, with particular emphasis on how they relate to public health. Finally, we look at the role of the public health professional in emergency preparedness—from designing policy to participating in disaster response—and explore potential careers in the field.

Part II begins to characterize the problems that require preparedness on the part of the public health community. Chapter 2 covers threats from biological, chemical, nuclear, and radiological weapons. We define these threats and review the history of use—both intentional and accidental. The chapter then looks at how the current threat from weapons of mass destruction (WMDs) is evaluated and returns to the role of the public health community in responding to WMD. Chapter 3 discusses threats from naturally occurring disease and natural disasters: the historical impact of disease and natural disaster on homeland and national security, preparedness activities around the threat of naturally occurring diseases, evaluation of the current threat from disease and disasters, and the public health and foreign policy response to these threats.

Part III moves from definitions and threat characterization to a review of the infrastructure, primarily on the federal level, that has emerged in the past decade to address public health preparedness. Chapter 4 focuses on the immediate response to September 11, 2001, and the 9/11 Commission findings. We review the National Strategy for Homeland Security and the offices and organizations that were created in the aftermath of 9/11. This chapter also introduces the reader to the intelligence community. Chapter 5 presents the preparedness plans that were created in response to evolving threats. We look at the National Response Framework—with particular emphasis on public health and medical response components, the National Incident Management System, and specific plans for public health emergencies. Finally, Chapter 6 presents the legislation, regulations, and policy guidance that have emerged to address public health preparedness and to mitigate the threats of WMD, naturally occurring disease, and other disasters.

Part IV of the book is generally concerned with solving problems, and it includes a variety of approaches the community has taken to address biological threats, along with the challenges of each approach. Chapter 7 explores biosecurity: defining the dual-use dilemma, determining how biosecurity is used to minimize the threat, examining the role of the life sciences community in establishing codes of conduct and self-policing scientific publications, reviewing pathogen security efforts, and examining synthetic biology as a threat to security. In Chapter 8, we look at the research agenda and which agencies are engaged in supporting basic scientific research that directly relates to biological threats. We also look at the enterprise that has been built to support the development of medical countermeasures and at the proliferation of biosafety level 3 and level 4 laboratories.

Chapter 9 focuses on the role of treaties in prevention of WMD and how international agreements have been used to address public health threats. Chapter 10 concentrates on the challenges associated with investigating an alleged use event and on making an attribution assessment. We explain microbial forensics, present the case study of a domestic investigation of alleged biological weapons use, and discuss the international mechanisms available for investigating suspected chemical and biological weapons use. This chapter also explores the relationship between the Federal Bureau of Investigation and the public health community, particularly as it pertains to criminal and epidemiological investigations.

In Chapter 11, we turn our attention to biosurveillance and discuss the domestic and international surveillance programs, as well as the federal entities, tasked with and engaged in these efforts. Chapter 12 provides several case studies of public health preparedness and response. We look at preparedness activities around avian influenza (H5N1); response activities around pandemic influenza (H1N1); and response mechanisms for natural disasters, including Hurricane Katrina and the Haiti earthquake. The final chapter, Chapter 13, takes the reader from the local preparedness level to global governance of disease. This chapter looks at the role of local preparedness activities, quarantine as part of preparedness and response, and global governance as it pertains to infectious diseases and public health emergencies of international concern.

This book is designed to give the reader an appreciation of the complexity of issues that must be considered by public health professionals in designing preparedness and response plans, policies, regulations, and legislation. I hope readers will better understand the essential role of the public health community in preparing for and responding to security threats.

Acknowledgments

This book is based on a class I teach at The George Washington University School of Public Health and Health Services—a class I inherited in 2006 from Brian Kamoie. So I first thank Brian for his foresight and efforts in designing this class and for trusting me to build on the foundation he provided. I thank the class for their helpful comments on earlier drafts of this book. I thank my colleagues for their support while I worked on this book, and I thank my team of research assistants without whom I would be lost, including Sarah Elrod, Jacqueline Miller, Adeela Khan, Jordan Chapman, and Daniel Bachmann. Most important, I thank my family—Matt, Olivia, and Benjamin—for their love and support.

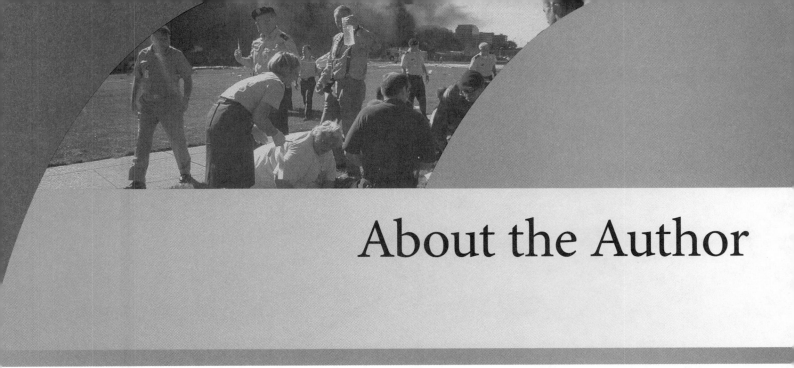

About the Author

Rebecca Katz, PhD, MPH, is an assistant professor of health policy and emergency medicine at The George Washington University School of Public Health and Health Services. Her research is focused on public health preparedness and the interface between infectious diseases and national security. Since 2007, the primary focus of her research has been on the domestic and global implementation of the Revised International Health Regulations. She previously worked on biological warfare counterproliferation at the Defense Intelligence Agency, was an Intelligence Research Fellow at the Center for Strategic Intelligence Research in the Joint Military Intelligence College, and spent several years as a public health consultant for The Lewin Group. Since 2004, Dr. Katz has been a consultant to the Department of State, working on issues related to the Biological Weapons Convention, avian and pandemic influenza, and disease surveillance. She is the co-editor of the 2nd edition of the *Encyclopedia of Bioterrorism Defense*, and author or co-author of more than 30 papers, book chapters, and policy briefs. Dr. Katz received her undergraduate degree in political science and economics from Swarthmore College, an MPH from Yale University, and a PhD in public affairs from Princeton University.

Abbreviations

AI	avian influenza		CREATE	Center for Risk and Economic Analysis of Terrorism Events
ALERT	Center of Excellence for Awareness and Location of Explosives—Related Threats		CRI	Cities Readiness Initiative
APHIS	Animal and Plant Health Inspection Service		CS	chlorobenzylidenemalononitrile
ARS	acute radiation syndrome		CTR	Cooperative Threat Reduction
ASPH	Association of Schools of Public Health		CW	chemical warfare/chemical weapons
ASPR	Assistant Secretary for Preparedness and Response		CWC	Chemical Weapons Convention
			CWS	Chemical Warfare Service
BARDA	Biomedical Advanced Research and Development Authority		DEA	Drug Enforcement Agency
			DHHS	Department of Health and Human Services
BEP	Biological Engagement Program		DHS	Department of Homeland Security
BSL	biosafety level		DIA	Defense Intelligence Agency
BT	bioterrorism		DMAT	Disaster Medical Assistance Team
BW	biological warfare/biological weapons		DNI	Director of National Intelligence
BWC	Biological and Toxin Weapons Convention		DoD	Department of Defense
C2I	Center of Excellence in Command, Control and Interoperability		DOS	Department of State
			DTRA	Defense Threat Reduction Agency
CAMRA	Center for Advancing Microbial Risk Assessment		EEE	Eastern Equine Encephalitis
CBRN	chemical, biological, radiological, and nuclear		EIS	Epidemic Intelligence Service
			EO	Executive Order
CBRNE	chemical, biological, radiological, nuclear, and explosive		ESF	Emergency Support Function
			FAA	Federal Aviation Administration
CDC	Centers for Disease Control and Prevention		FAZD	National Center for Foreign Animal and Zoonotic Disease Defense
CIA	Central Intelligence Agency			
CN	chloroacetophenone		FBI	Federal Bureau of Investigation
COE	Centers of Excellence		FDA	Food and Drug Administration
CONUS	Continental United States		FEMA	Federal Emergency Management Agency

FSU	Former Soviet Union
GDD	Global Disease Detection
GOARN	Global Outbreak Alert and Response Network
HSEEP	Homeland Security Exercise and Evaluation Program
HSPD	Homeland Security Presidential Directive
HUMINT	human intelligence
IA	Office of Intelligence and Analysis (DHS)
IAEA	International Atomic Energy Agency
IARPA	Intelligence Advanced Research Projects Activity
IBC	Institutional Biosafety Committee
IC	intelligence community
IHR	International Health Regulations
IO	international organization
IOM	Institute of Medicine
IMINT	imagery intelligence
INR	Bureau of Intelligence and Research (DOS)
IRF	Integrated Research Facility
MASINT	Measurement and Signature Intelligence
MDR-TB	multiple-drug-resistant tuberculosis
MIC	methyl isocyanate
MPH	Masters in Public Health
MSEHPA	Model State Emergency Health Powers Act
NAS	National Academies of Science
NBACC	National Biodefense Analysis and Countermeasure Center
NBIC	National Biosurveillance Integration Center
NCFPT	National Center for Food Protection and Defense
NCI	National Cancer Institute
NCIX	National Counterintelligence Executive
NCPC	National Counterproliferation Center
NCTC	National Counterterrorism Center
NDMS	National Disaster Medical System
NGA	National Geospatial-Intelligence Agency
NGO	nongovernmental organization
NHSS	National Health Security Strategy
NIAID	National Institute of Allergy and Infectious Diseases
NIC	National Intelligence Council
NIC	National Integration Center
NIH	National Institutes of Health

NIMS	National Incident Management System
NIEHS	National Institute of Environmental Health Sciences
NINDS	National Institute of Neurological Disorders and Stroke
NIU	National Intelligence University
NORAD	North American Aerospace Defense Command
NORTHCOM	Northern Command
NPS	National Pharmaceutical Stockpile
NRF	National Response Framework
NRO	National Reconnaissance Office
NRP	National Response Plan
NSA	National Security Agency
NSABB	National Science Advisory Board for Biosecurity
NSD	National Security Directive
NSDD	National Security Decision Directive
NSPD	National Security Presidential Directive
NTSCOE	National Transportation Security Center of Excellence
OSINT	Open Source Intelligence
OSTP	Office of Science and Technology Policy
OTA	Office of Technology Assessment
PACER	National Center of the Study for Preparedness and Catastrophic Event Response
PAHPA	Pandemic and All-Hazards Preparedness Act
PDD	Presidential Decision Directive
PEPFAR	U.S. President's Emergency Plan for AIDS Relief
PHEIC	Public Health Emergency of International Concern
PHEMCE	Public Health Emergency Medical Countermeasures Enterprise
PHS	Public Health Service
PNAS	Proceedings of the National Academy of Sciences
PPD	Presidential Policy Directive
PREP	Public Readiness and Emergency Preparedness Act
PS	chloropicrin
RCE	Regional Center of Excellence [for biodefense and emerging infectious diseases]
SARS	severe acute respiratory syndrome
SEPA	Smallpox Emergency Personnel Protection Act

SIGINT	Signals Intelligence
SNS	Strategic National Stockpile
SSC	Special Security Center
START	National Consortium for the Study of Terrorism and Responses to Terrorism
T2	trichothecene mycotoxin
TB	tuberculosis
TCL	Target Capabilities List
TECHINT	Technical Intelligence
UNSCR	United Nations Security Council Resolution
UNSGM	United Nations Secretary General's Mechanism
USAID	United States Agency for International Development
USAMRIID	U.S. Army Medical Research Institute for Infectious Diseases
USA PATRIOT	Uniting and Strengthening America by Providing Appropriate Tools Required to Intercept and Obstruct Terrorism

USC	United States Code
USDA	U.S. Department of Agriculture
USPS	U.S. Postal Service
UTL	universal task list
UTMB	University of Texas Medical Branch
VEE	Venezuelan Equine Encephalitis
WEE	Western Equine Encephalitis
WHA	World Health Assembly
WHO	World Health Organization
WMD	weapon of mass destruction
WRS	War Research Service
WWI	World War I
WWII	World War II
XDR-TB	extremely drug-resistant tuberculosis

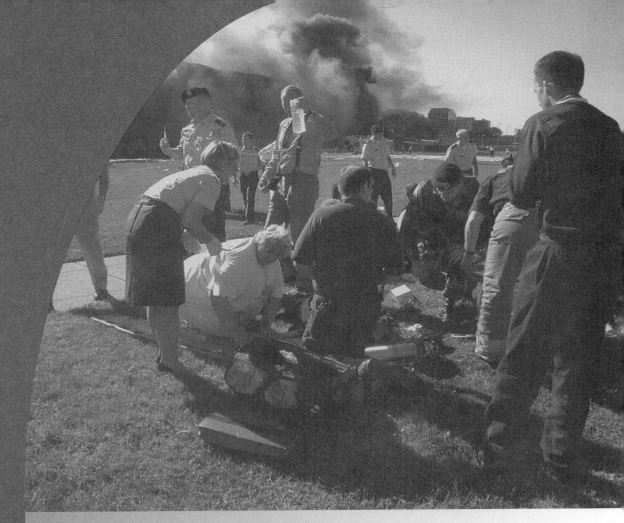

PART I

Background of the Field

CHAPTER 1

Introduction to Public Health Preparedness

LEARNING OBJECTIVES

By the end of this chapter, the reader will be able to:

- Define public health preparedness and understand the scope of events that can lead to a public health emergency.
- Identify the difference between homeland and national security.
- Understand the role of the public health professional in emergency preparedness and response activities.
- Be familiar with the types of careers available to public health professionals in preparedness.

BOX 1-1 Preamble to the Constitution of the United States of America

We the People of the United States, in Order to form a more perfect Union, establish Justice, insure domestic Tranquility, provide for the common defense, promote the general Welfare, and secure the Blessings of Liberty to ourselves and our Posterity, do ordain and establish this Constitution for the United States of America.

INTRODUCTION

The Preamble to the Constitution of the United States of America lays the groundwork for creation of the nation and for the basic responsibilities of the federal government. (See **Box 1-1**.) Among these responsibilities are to "provide for the common defense" and "promote the general welfare." Public health preparedness, as a subdiscipline of public health, strives to address these two fundamental components of a government's responsibility to its population.

The notions of both homeland security and national security are paramount to public health preparedness. Before we define public health preparedness, let us start with what exactly "provide for the common defense" means.

NATIONAL SECURITY

Political scientists have long debated what exactly defines *national security*. The concept means different things to different people.[1(pp 41–56)] Some see it as policies, including diplomatic, economic, and military power, enacted by governments in

order to ensure the survival and safety of the State.[1(pp 41–56)] Others define it as safeguarding territorial integrity and national independence—basically, the existence of the State.[1(pp 41–56)] George Kennan wrote that national security is "the continued ability of this country to pursue its internal life without serious interference."[1(pp 52–53)] The reoccurring theme within all discussions of national security, however, is the extent to which an individual is willing to sacrifice freedom in exchange for security, and the balance between security and liberty.

The most extreme position regarding national security is that it does not matter if the threat to security comes from within or from outside the nation. Citizens will look to the State for protection against all types of threats. In exchange, the State can ask anything of that citizen, short of his/her life. (See **Box 1-2**.) For most people, and particularly for those in the United States, a more balanced perspective of security and personal liberty prevails. While U.S. citizens want to be

---

BOX 1-2 **Excerpt from *Leviathan* (1651) by Thomas Hobbes**

Without security provided for by the state, there is . . .
". . . *continual fear, and danger of violent death; and the life of man, solitary, poor, nasty, brutish, and short.*"

---

protected from threats and support the government in doing so, they want it to be done in such a way that they are able to retain personal freedoms and liberties.

HOMELAND SECURITY

The founding fathers penned the argument that the Constitution would protect U.S. citizens against conflict at home and that geography would protect the nation from conflict abroad.[2] The basic belief was that no threat would reach our borders; the oceans would protect us from conflict on our shores. As history has proven, however, geography cannot protect us from all external threats, particularly from terrorist actors.

After the terrorist attacks on September 11, 2001, the nation, for the first time, began to speak collectively about "homeland security." The Department of Defense (DoD) defines *homeland security* as "the prevention, preemption, deterrence of, and defense against aggression targeted at US territory, sovereignty, domestic population, and infrastructure, as well as the management of the consequences of such aggression and other domestic emergencies."[3(p 24)] Other definitions vary slightly,[4(p 2),5(p 11)] but, at the core, homeland security is about preventing disasters and attacks on the United States (primarily the continental United States, also known as "CONUS") and minimizing damage through appropriate preparations and rapid recovery.

Homeland Defense

Homeland defense is a component of homeland security. *Homeland Defense* is "the protection of U.S. sovereignty, territory, domestic population, and critical defense infrastructure against external threats or aggression."[6] Broadly, this means everything from national missile defense to critical infrastructure protection. The concepts of preparedness and response, however, are included in "security" and not in "defense."

PUBLIC HEALTH PREPAREDNESS

Public health preparedness, like homeland security, is a term that represents concerns and actions that have occurred throughout history. The term itself, however, and the field devoted to thinking about, preparing for, and mobilizing resources to respond to public health emergencies are relatively new. The field is so new that it is still struggling to define itself and to establish core competencies for professionals working in the area.

The Association of Schools of Public Health (ASPH) defines public health preparedness as "a combination of comprehensive planning, infrastructure building, capacity building, communication, training and evaluation that increase public health response effectiveness and efficiency in response to infectious disease outbreaks, bioterrorism and emerging health threats."[7(p 5)] In 2007, a group at the RAND Corporation, however, proposed a definition, providing a slightly broader characterization of the field:

> [P]ublic health emergency preparedness . . . is the capability of the public health and health care systems, communities, and individuals, to prevent, protect against, quickly respond to, and recover from health emergencies, particularly those whose scale, timing, or unpredictability threatens to overwhelm routine capabilities. Preparedness involves a coordinated and continuous process of planning and implementation that relies on measuring performance and taking corrective action.[8(p S9)]

This definition raises the question, What exactly is a public health emergency? According to the RAND definition, it is an event "whose scale, timing, or unpredictability threatens to overwhelm routine capabilities." These types of events fit into four basic categories:

1. Natural disasters, such as hurricanes, earthquakes, floods, or fires.
2. Man-made environmental disasters, such as oil spills.
3. Natural epidemics or pandemics, which may involve a novel, emerging infectious disease; a reemerging agent; or a previously controlled disease.
4. The intentional or accidental release of a chemical, biological, radiological, or nuclear (CBRN) agent.

For any of these four categories of events to be classified as a public health emergency, it is not just enough for the event to occur, but it also must pose a high probability of large-scale morbidity, mortality, or a risk of future harm.[9(p 11)]

Yet another category of public health emergency exists, as defined by the legally binding World Health Organization's International Health Regulations (2005), which will be discussed in more detail in Chapter 9. This international agreement defines a public health emergency of international concern (PHEIC) as "[A]n extraordinary event which is determined . . . to constitute a public health risk to other States through the international spread of disease and to potentially require a coordinated international response."[10] Such an emergency can involve any of the preceding four types of public health events, as long as it has the potential to cross borders.

Some public health issues that have been called "emergencies" do not meet the criteria of any of these definitions. The obesity epidemic[11] or the prevalence of breast cancer,[12(pp 2282–2283)] for example, may be "public health crises," but they are not considered emergencies within the purview of public health preparedness.*

Our understanding of the types of events that constitute public health emergencies has changed over time. Later chapters of this book will focus on the evolving threats, examples of how the public health community has addressed these types of emergencies, and what we have learned from our experiences to date.

The responsibility of the public health community to prepare for and address these acute health emergencies is extensive. **Box 1-3** summarizes some of the principal components

---

BOX 1-3 Components of Public Health Preparedness and Community Preparedness

1. **Health risk assessment:** identification of "hazards and vulnerabilities . . . that will form the basis for planning."

2. **Legal climate:** identification and amendment, as necessary, of legal authority and liability barriers to effective monitoring, prevention, and response to public health emergencies.

3. **Roles and responsibilities:** clearly defining, assigning, and testing responsibilities with all potential parties involved in preparedness and response.

4. **Incident command system:** developing, testing, and improving response capabilities using an integrated system at all levels (e.g., local, state, federal, and tribal).

5. **Public engagement:** ensuring the public is informed, engaged, and mobilized to be active participants in preparedness activities.

6. **Epidemiology functions:** maintaining and improving surveillance systems for detection of potential emergencies and investigation of events.

7. **Laboratory functions:** maintaining and improving laboratory testing and detection of public health hazards.

8. **Countermeasures and mitigation strategies:** developing, testing, and improving distribution of medical countermeasures and community mitigation strategies, including isolation, quarantine, and social distancing.

9. **Mass health care:** developing, testing, and improving the healthcare system's ability to provide for large numbers of affected people.

10. **Public information and communication:** developing and improving the capability to provide timely and appropriate information about public health emergencies.

11. **Workforce:** developing and maintaining a public health workforce to respond appropriately to all public health emergencies.

Note: Original work by RAND also includes the following as components of a prepared community: a robust supply chain, leadership, testing operational capabilities, performance management, and financial tracking.

Source: Nelson C, Lurie N, Wasserman J, Zakowski S. Conceptualizing and Defining Public Health Emergency Preparedness. *American Journal of Public Health.* 2007;97(S1):S10.

---

* Interestingly, recent literature has started to link obesity to national security because the prevalence of overweight youth is affecting the ability of the United States to recruit fit personnel for the armed forces.[13]

of public health preparedness, particularly from the perspective of the "prepared community." This list of 11 major components is adapted from research conducted by Nelson and colleagues.

DEVELOPING THE PUBLIC HEALTH PREPAREDNESS WORKFORCE: CHARGE AND CAREERS

In December 2006, Congress passed the Pandemic and All-Hazards Preparedness Act (known as PAHPA, pronounced "papa"), which reauthorized and built upon the Public Health Security and Bioterrorism Preparedness and Response Act of 2002 (also known as the Bioterrorism Act) and is scheduled to be reauthorized in late 2011. Among other things, PAHPA called for the development of a public health workforce versed in preparedness and public health security capabilities, as shown in **Box 1-4**. It requires curricula to be developed and calls for the facilitation of competency-based training in pub-

lic health preparedness within schools of public health and other institutions.

In an effort to fulfill PAHPA's mandate, the Association of Schools of Public Health—in response to a request from the U.S. Centers for Disease Control and Prevention (CDC)—is developing model core competencies in public health preparedness and response to be released in late 2011. ASPH efforts are targeted at public health workers who have 10 years of experience or 5 years with a master's in public health (MPH) or higher degree.[14]

In today's security climate, it is important for many different types of public health professionals, at every level of government and the private sector, with diverse knowledge and expertise, to be versed in public health preparedness. When a public health emergency occurs, it affects the entire public health and medical system. Everyone from laboratory technicians to clinicians to program managers may be affected.

BOX 1-4 Pandemic and All-Hazards Preparedness Act (PAHPA) of 2006. Section 304: Core Education and Training

TITLE III—ALL-HAZARDS MEDICAL SURGE CAPACITY
SEC. 304. CORE EDUCATION AND TRAINING.

(d) Centers for Public Health Preparedness; Core Curricula and Training—

(1) IN GENERAL—The Secretary may establish at accredited schools of public health, Centers for Public Health Preparedness (hereafter referred to in this section as the "Centers").

(2) ELIGIBILITY—To be eligible to receive an award under this subsection to establish a Center, an accredited school of public health shall agree to conduct activities consistent with the requirements of this subsection.

(3) CORE CURRICULA—The Secretary, in collaboration with the Centers and other public or private entities shall establish core curricula based on established competencies leading to a 4-year bachelor's degree, a graduate degree, a combined bachelor and master's degree, or a certificate program, for use by each Center. The Secretary shall disseminate such curricula to other accredited schools of public health and other health professions schools determined appropriate by the Secretary, for voluntary use by such schools.

(4) CORE COMPETENCY-BASED TRAINING PROGRAM—The Secretary, in collaboration with the Centers and other public or private entities shall facilitate the development of a competency-based training program to train public health practitioners. The Centers shall use such training program to train public health practitioners. The Secretary shall disseminate such training program to other accredited schools of public health, health professions schools, and other public or private entities as determined by the Secretary, for voluntary use by such entities.

(5) CONTENT OF CORE CURRICULA AND TRAINING PROGRAM—The Secretary shall ensure that the core curricula and training program established pursuant to this subsection respond to the needs of State, local, and tribal public health authorities and integrate and emphasize essential public health security capabilities consistent with section 2802(b)(2).

Jobs in Public Health Preparedness

Merely 10 years after being defined as a subdiscipline, trained professionals in public health preparedness are now sought after by a multitude of organizations and agencies.

- *Private sector:* Think tanks, consulting firms, private industry, and government contractors hire public health professionals who specialize in preparedness. These jobs include operational planning for private companies, strategic planning for the pharmaceutical industry, and policy analysis and training to support both government entities and clinical operations.
- *State and local government:* Just about every state and local health department now has dedicated staff for preparedness and emergency planning. In addition, state and local departments of emergency management, agriculture, commerce, and transportation, as well as legal support offices, may also employ public health preparedness experts, which again demonstrates the necessity of diverse expertise.
- *Federal government:* As we will learn throughout this text, the federal government is heavily involved in public health preparedness, requiring skilled professionals to work not just at the Department of Health and Human Services but also at the Departments of State, Agriculture, Defense, Treasury, Justice, and Homeland Security and within the intelligence community and the U.S. Agency for International Development.
- *Academia:* Researchers are needed to further the field of preparedness, and informed professors are required for curriculum development and training of students and midcareer professionals.
- *International organizations:* Nongovernmental organizations (NGOs) and formal international organizations (IOs), such as those that are part of the United Nations, are engaged in public health preparedness activities. These include everything from disaster management to refugee health to public health aspects of the Biological Weapons Convention and implementation of the International Health Regulations.

In all, a great deal of work needs to be accomplished, and the need for smart, energetic, and enthusiastic people is great. The world can always use more strong public health professionals and, specifically, public health professionals who can contribute to emergency preparedness and response.

KEY WORDS

Public health preparedness
National security
Homeland security
Homeland defense
Workforce
Pandemic and All Hazards Preparedness Act (PAHPA)
Core competencies
Community preparedness

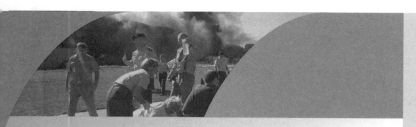

Discussion Questions

1. Is public health preparedness the same as national preparedness? Is public health preparedness well defined? Can it be operationalized?

2. What types of emergency events require a public health role?

3. What types of public health emergencies require planning for underserved populations and how might such planning be incorporated into preparedness activities?

4. What is the difference between national and homeland security?

5. During a public health emergency, what types of organizations, entities, businesses, and officials will have a stake in response and recovery operations?

6. From the list of 11 components of public health preparedness, which 3 do you think are most important and should be prioritized? Why?

REFERENCES

1. Bergen P, Garrett L. The Princeton Project on National Security Report of the Working Group on State Security and Transnational Threats. 2006. Available at: http://www.princeton.edu/~ppns/conferences/reports/fall/SSTT.pdf. Accessed May 27, 2010.

2. Hamilton A. *The Federalist No. 8, The Consequences of Hostilities Between the States.* November 20, 1787.

3. Advanced Materials and Processes Technology Information Analysis Center. Homeland Security vs. Homeland Defense. Is there a difference? *The AMPTIAC Quarterly.* February 2003;6(4). Available at: http://ammtiac.alionscience.com/pdf/AMPQ6_4.pdf. Accessed May 18, 2011.

4. Office of Homeland Security. *National Strategy for Homeland Security.* July 2002. Available at: http://www.dhs.gov/xlibrary/assets/nat_strat_hls.pdf. Accessed May 18, 2011.

5. Kettl DF. *The States and Homeland Security, Building the Missing Link.* The Century Foundation. 2003. Available at: http://www.tcf.org/Publications/HomelandSecurity/kettl.pdf. Accessed May 18, 2011.

6. United States Department of Defense. DoD 101, An Introductory Overview of the Department of Defense. Available at: http://www.defense.gov/pubs/dod101/dod101.html. Accessed May 30, 2010.

7. Association of Schools of Public Health Core Curricula Working Group. *Practical Implications, Approaches, Opportunities and Challenges of a Preparedness Core Curricula in Accredited Schools of Public Health.* Available at: http://www.asph.org/UserFiles/finalcorecurriculawhitepaper1.pdf. Accessed May 18, 2011.

8. Nelson C, Lurie N, Wasserman J, Zakowski S. Conceptualizing and Defining Public Health Emergency Preparedness. *American Journal of Public Health.* 2007;97(S1):S9–S11.

9. The Center for Law and the Public's Health at Georgetown and Johns Hopkins Universities. *The Model State Emergency Health Powers Act.* December 21, 2001. Available at: http://www.publichealthlaw.net/MSEHPA/MSEHPA.pdf. Accessed May 18, 2011.

10. World Health Organization. *International Health Regulations* (2005) 2nd ed. 2008:Article I. Available at: http://whqlibdoc.who.int/publications/2008/9789241580410_eng.pdf. Accessed May 18, 2011.

11. Brown WV, Fujioka K, Wilson PWF, Woodworth KA. Obesity: Why Be Concerned? *The American Journal of Medicine.* April 2009;122(4A).

12. Harford J, Azavedo E, Fischietto M. Guideline Implementation for Breast Healthcare in Low- and Middle-Income Countries: Breast Healthcare Program Resource Allocation. *Cancer.* October 2008;113(S8):2282–2296.

13. Association of Schools of Public Health Preparedness and Response Core Competency Development Project Leadership Group. *Public Health Preparedness and Response Core Competency Development Project Tenets, Target Audience, and Performance Level.* 2010. Available at: http://www.asph.org/userfiles/PrepResponse-TenetsAudience.pdf. Accessed May 18, 2011.

14. Shalikashvili JM, Shelton H. The latest national security threat: obesity. *The Washington Post.* April 2010:A19. Available at: http://www.washingtonpost.com/wp-dyn/content/article/2010/04/29/AR2010042903669.html. Accessed May 18, 2011.

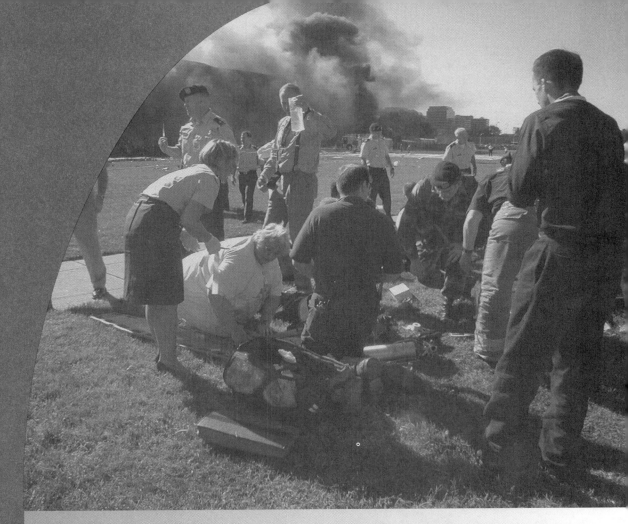

PART II

Defining the Problem: Potential Threats

CHAPTER 2

Threats from Biological, Chemical, Nuclear, and Radiological Weapons

LEARNING OBJECTIVES

By the end of this chapter, the reader will be able to:

- Define biological, chemical, radiological, and nuclear weapons.
- Understand the threats from and history of use of weapons of mass destruction.
- Characterize the current threat from weapons of mass destruction, specifically biological weapons, used by both state and nonstate actors.
- Identify the public health community's role in responding to weapons of mass destruction.

INTRODUCTION

In this chapter, we begin to explore and define the threats the public health community should be prepared to address. We begin with a focus on weapons of mass destruction (WMD), including chemical, biological, radiological, and nuclear (CBRN) weapons. While we will look at all of these types of weapons, our predominant focus will be on biological weapons because they are most directly linked to the public health and medical communities through detection, response, and recovery. However, for the public health and medical communities to be prepared for and to respond appropriately to these threats, they must work closely with communities that they may not have traditionally interacted with, particularly the security and defense communities—including law enforcement, military entities, the intelligence community, and the rest of the national and homeland security infrastructure. These communities, and specific interactions, will be discussed in more detail later in the book. Here, we present the WMD threats. We look first at chemical, then nuclear and radiological threats, and then focus more extensively on the details of biological

weapons. The majority of this chapter and the rest of this text will center on the biological threat because this threat has the strongest links to public health preparedness.

CHEMICAL THREATS

Article II, paragraph 1, of the Chemical Weapons Convention (CWC), defines chemical weapons as one of the following, either in combination or separately:

> (a) Toxic chemicals and their precursors, except where intended for purposes not prohibited under this Convention, as long as the types and quantities are consistent with such purposes;
>
> (b) Munitions and devices, specifically designed to cause death or other harm through the toxic properties of those toxic chemicals specified in subparagraph (a), which would be released as a result of the employment of such munitions and devices;
>
> (c) Any equipment specifically designed for use directly in connection with the employment of munitions and devices specified in subparagraph (b).[1]

In general, chemical warfare is the use of a chemical substance to directly harm or kill humans, plants,* or animals. Chemical agents are nonliving, manufactured chemicals.

---

* It is worth noting that the Chemical Weapons Convention does not include chemicals that harm plants. There is some debate over whether defoliants and other chemicals used against plants should be considered chemical weapons under international legal regimes.

They tend to be highly toxic and can enter the body through inhalation or through the skin. Adding to the complexity of treatment, illness or death can come within minutes of exposure or take as long as several hours.[2] As described in **Box 2-1**, there are four main categories of chemical warfare agents: blister (e.g., mustard gas), blood (e.g., cyanide), choking (e.g., chlorine), and nerve (e.g., sarin). In addition, a class, termed *riot control agents*, produce temporary, usually nonfatal, irritation of the skin, eyes, and respiratory tract. Riot control agents, often known as "tear gas," include chloroacetophenone (CN), chlorobenzylidenemalononitrile (CS), and chloropicrin (PS). The Chemical Weapons Convention and the U.S. government do not consider this class of agents to be chemical weapons. Other nations, however, disagree.[3]

TOXINS

Toxins are nonliving poisons produced by living entities, such as plants, fungi, insects, and animals. Because they are chemical by-products of biological agents, they occupy a conceptual gray area between chemical and biological weapons. The Biological Weapons Convention covers toxins, as does the Chemical Weapons Convention—or at least some toxins. This is another area where, for the purposes of arms control and legal international obligations, countries do not always agree on how toxins should be categorized.

BOX 2-1 Types of Chemical Agents

- *Nerve agents*—primarily act on the nervous system, causing seizures and death. Examples of this category include sarin, VX, tabun, and soman. This category also includes fourth-generation chemical weapons, known as Novichok agents, which are thought to be much more lethal than VX.
- *Blister agents, or vesicants*—primarily cause irritation of the skin and mucous membrane. Examples of this category include mustard gas and arsenical Lewisite.
- *Choking agents, or pulmonary toxicants*—primarily cause damage to the lungs, including pulmonary edema and hemorrhage. Examples include phosgene, diphosgene, and chlorine.
- *Blood agents*— in high doses, primarily cause seizures and respiratory and cardiac failure. Examples include hydrogen cyanide and cyanogen cyanide.

History

In April 1915, during World War I, in Ypres, France, the German army attacked the French with chlorine gas, marking the first large-scale use of chemical weapons during warfare. Several months later, in September 1915, the British used chlorine gas against the Germans at the Battle of Loos. This was followed in June 1918 by the first use of chemical warfare by the United States. It was clear that by the end of World War I, all sides were actively using the chemical weapons.[4] **Figure 2-1** shows soldiers in World War I suffering from the effects of chemical warfare.

Many nations continued to utilize chemical warfare throughout the 20th century, including the British use of Adamsite (a vomiting agent) against the Bolsheviks during the Russian Civil War, Spanish use of chemical weapons against rebels in Morocco in the 1920s, Italian use of mustard gas against Ethiopians in 1936, and the Nazi's use of hydrocyanic acid for the mass extermination of Jews and other concentration camp prisoners during World War II.[5]

During the Vietnam War, the United States used defoliants, such as dioxin, also known as "Agent Orange," as well as other normally nonlethal agents. The United States does not consider defoliants to be chemical weapons; therefore, it does not consider this use to be chemical warfare. High levels of morbidity and mortality from those exposed to the agents, though, have led to large research efforts and calls by many that this was, in fact, chemical warfare.[6,7]

While most of the cited examples of chemical weapons use have been large-scale warfare incidents, these agents have also been used throughout history as assassination tools.[8] One particularly illustrative example was the 1979 assassination of a Bulgarian exile, named Georgie Markov, described in **Box 2-2**.

Another example of the offensive use of chemical agents comes from the doomsday cult Aum Shinrikyo, based in Japan. On March 20, 1995, Aum Shinrikyo released sarin gas into the Tokyo subway system. Twelve people died, approximately 50 were severely injured, and almost 1,000 suffered temporary vision problems.[9] More than 5,500 people, however, sought medical attention, swarming area hospitals and testing public health capacities. This chemical weapons use event highlighted the importance of emergency preparedness, especially in the area of hospital surge capacity.

In addition to intentional releases of chemical agents, the accidental releases of agents have also posed significant challenges to public health and medical systems worldwide and have adversely affected the health of populations. For example, in 1981, cooking oil was accidentally adulterated with industrial rapeseed oil and distributed throughout southern

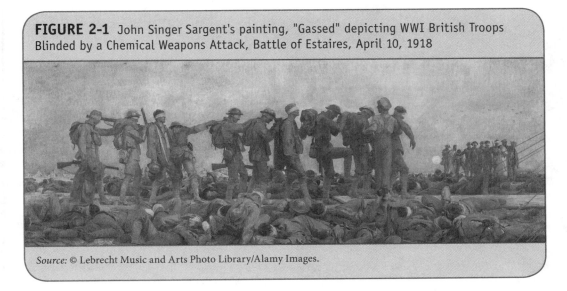

FIGURE 2-1 John Singer Sargent's painting, "Gassed" depicting WWI British Troops Blinded by a Chemical Weapons Attack, Battle of Estaires, April 10, 1918

Source: © Lebrecht Music and Arts Photo Library/Alamy Images.

Europe. More than 15,000 people became sick, and 203 died after people consumed the contaminated oil.[10(p xi)]

In some instances, the release of chemical agents may not have been entirely accidental, but one assumes that the public health consequences were unintentional. In 2006, a Panamanian-flag, Greek-owned, Swiss oil company–chartered tanker, the *Probo Koala*, avoiding European disposal fees, carried more than 500 tons of petrochemical waste to Côte d'Ivoire, which was then dumped by a local contractor in more than 12 different sites around Abidjan. Fifteen people died as a result of exposure to this toxic waste, 69 were hospitalized, and more than 100,000 sought medical treatment,[11] easily overwhelming the existing public health and medical infrastructures.[12] **Figure 2-2** shows a worker involved in trying to clean up the toxic waste.

Unfortunately, these types of exposures to chemical agents are not infrequent. On May 29, 2010, a worker at a scrapyard in Nigeria tried to cut a gas cylinder into pieces,

---

BOX 2-2 Assassination by Ricin

In 1978, a Bulgarian exile, named Georgie Markov, was waiting for a bus in London. A man poked him with the tip of an umbrella, apologized, and got into a taxi. Four days later Markov was dead.

Ten days prior to this incident, another Bulgarian exile, Vladimir Kostov, was shot in the back in Paris, and when he turned around, he witnessed someone running away with an umbrella. This particular umbrella had been adapted and rebuilt into a makeshift gun that fired ricin pellets from its tip. After learning of Markov's death, Kostov sought medical attention immediately. A doctor removed the pellet that had lodged in his back. Fortunately, the ricin that was contained within the pellet had not fully expelled into his bloodstream. The doctor successfully removed it and confirmed the presence of ricin; Kostov survived the incident.

One of the reasons ricin was such an effective assassination tool against Markov was that it was virtually impossible to detect what was killing him and authorities could have done little even if it was identified. Ricin, a poison extracted from castor beans, prevents cells in the body from making proteins; without proteins, cells die, which can eventually lead to death. Once someone is exposed, it can take up to 6 to 8 hours for symptoms to occur, depending on the route of exposure, and death can occur rapidly within 36 to 72 hours. The symptoms of ricin exposure include respiratory distress if inhaled, vomiting and diarrhea if ingested, and redness and pain of skin and eyes if absorbed through skin. There is no available antidote thus far, and the only treatment is supportive medical care.

Source: Centers for Disease Control and Prevention. Facts about Ricin. *Emergency Preparedness and Response.* March 5, 2008. Available at: http://www.bt.cdc.gov/agent/ricin/facts.asp. Accessed July 8, 2010; Carus WS. *Bioterrorism and biocrimes: The illicit use of biological agents since 1900.* Center for Counterproliferation Research, National Defense University, 2001.

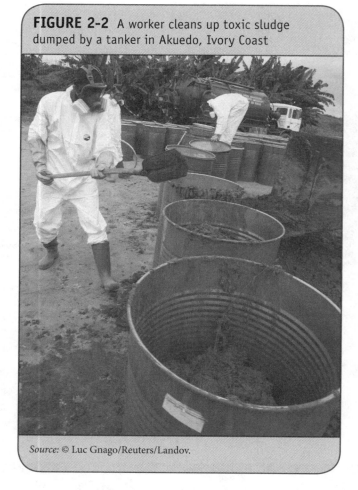

FIGURE 2-2 A worker cleans up toxic sludge dumped by a tanker in Akuedo, Ivory Coast

Source: © Luc Gnago/Reuters/Landov.

resulting in an explosion that released a cloud of chlorine gas into the air, sickening 300 people, who eventually required medical treatment.[13]

The largest chemical agent accidental exposure took place on December 3, 1984, in Bhopal, India. A Union Carbide pesticide plant released 40 tons of methyl isocyanate (MIC) gas into the air in the middle of the night. Nearly 4,000 people died instantly, and the total number of deaths is estimated to be between 15,000 and 22,000. A total of 500,000 people were exposed, and as many as 120,000 continue to suffer detrimental health effects.[14]

Accidents that expose populations to chemical agents can occur anywhere, including the United States. For example, a community in Graniteville, South Carolina, was left with 9 dead and 250 injured after a train carrying toxic chemicals, including chlorine gas, crashed. Accidents such as this, as well as the additional events listed in **Table 2-1**, remind us that all public health communities, regardless of location, must have a level of awareness regarding preparedness for a variety of potential public health emergencies, including the need to know how to respond to an emergency.

NUCLEAR AND RADIOLOGICAL THREATS

Nuclear Weapons

A nuclear weapon that involves fission (the splitting of atoms), like the bomb that the United States dropped on Hiroshima, Japan, or the devastating weapons created and stockpiled by a small number of nations since, leaves a limited role for the public health community. If released, such weapons would instantly destroy people, buildings and anything else in the vicinity. A public health response would not be needed because the chances of survival would be minimal. The explosion, however, would leave behind large amounts of radioactivity. We discuss the challenge of radioactivity next.

Radiological Threats

A radiological event is an explosion or other release of radioactivity. Such an event might be caused by any of the following: a simple, nonexplosive radiological device; an improvised nuclear device designed to release large amounts of radiation with a large blast radius (such as a "suitcase bomb"); a dispersal device that combines explosive materials and radioactive material (such as a "dirty bomb"); or sabotage or other damage to a nuclear reactor that results in the release of radiation.[15]

Even a small dose of radiation can cause some detectable changes in blood. Large doses of radiation can lead to acute radiation syndrome (ARS). First signs of ARS are typically nausea, vomiting, headache, diarrhea, and some loss of white blood cells. These signs are followed by hair loss, damage to nerve cells and cells that line the digestive tract, and severe loss of white blood cells. The higher the dose of radiation, the less likely the person will survive. Those who do survive may take several weeks to 2 years to recover, and survivors may suffer from leukemia or other cancers.[16]

The public health implications of radiological exposure can be significant. In addition to all other functions, the public health community will be responsible for:

- Participating in shelter-in-place or evacuation decisions.
- Identifying exposed populations through surveillance activities.
- Conducting or assisting with environmental decontamination.
- Determining safety requirements for working in or near the site of the incident.
- Conducting near and long-term follow-up with exposed populations.[17]

To date, most radiological exposure has occurred via accidents. An often-cited event occurred in Goiânia, Brazil, in 1987. Two men were rummaging through an abandoned hos-

TABLE 2-1 Examples of Major Chemical Incidents (1974–2006)

Year	Location	Type of incident	Chemical(s) involved	Deaths	Injured	Evacuated
1974	Flixborough, United Kingdom	Chemical plant (explosion)	Cyclohexane 28	104	3,000	
1976	Seveso, Italy	Chemical plant (explosion)	Dioxin		193	226,000
1979	Novosibirsk, Russian Federation	Chemical plant (explosion)	Uncharacterized	300		
1981	Madrid, Spain	Foodstuff contamination (oil)	Uncharacterized	430	20,000	220,000
1982	Tacoa, Venezuela (Bolivarian Republic of)	Tank (explosion)	Fuel oil	153	20,000	40,000
1984	San Juanico, Mexico	Tank (explosion)	Liquified petroleum gas (LPG)	452	4,248	200,000
1984	Bhopal, India	Chemical plant (leak)	Methyl isocyanate	2,800	50,000	200,000
1992	Kwangju, Democratic People's Republic of Korea	Gas store (explosion)	LPG		163	20,000
1993	Bangkok, Thailand	Toy factory (fire)	Plastics	240	547	
1993	Remeios, Colombia	Spillage	Crude oil	430		
1996	Haiti	Poisoned medicine	Diethylene glycol	>60		
1998	Yaoundé, Cameroon	Transport accident	Petroleum products	220	130	
2000	Kinshasa, Democratic Republic of the Congo	Munitions depot (explosion)	Munitions	109	216	
2000	Enschede, Netherlands	Factory (explosion)	Fireworks	20	950	
2001	Toulouse, France	Factory (explosion)	Ammonium nitrate	30	>2,500	
2002	Lagos, Nigeria	Munitions depot (explosion)	Munitions	1,000		
2003	Gaoqiao, China	Gas well (release)	Hydrogen sulphide	240	9,000	64,000
2005	Huaian, China	Truck (release)	Chlorine	27	300	10,000
2005	Graniteville, United States of America	Train tanker (release)	Chlorine	9	250	5,400
2006	Abidjan, Côte d'Ivoire	Toxic waste	Hydrogen sulphide, mercaptans, sodium hydroxide	10	>100,000[a]	

[a] The number of consultations, not necessarily the number of people made directly ill.

Source: Modified from the World Health Organization. *The World Health Report 2007: A Safer Future—Global Public Health Security in the 21st Century,* 2007.

pital and found an old nuclear medicine source—a radioactive cesium-137 teletherapy head. They took it home, partially dismantled it, and eventually sold it to a scrapyard. The owner of the scrapyard discovered that the cesium capsule omitted a blue light; many came to see it, and children rubbed the material on their bodies to glow in the dark. Four people, in-cluding a young child, died from the exposure. Another 249 individuals suffered serious health consequences.[18]

The most serious radiation accidents have been associated with nuclear power plants. Sixty-three accidents have occurred at nuclear power plants, with the most serious occurring in Chernobyl, Ukraine. On April 26, 1986, at 1:23 a.m.,

Reactor 4 of the Chernobyl Nuclear Power Plant exploded, instantly killing three and sending a plume of radioactive fallout into the air, which eventually drifted over parts of the Soviet Union; eastern, western, and northern Europe; and eastern North America. Approximately 350,000 individuals had to be evacuated and resettled. Fifty-six people died as a direct result of the accident. Another 4,000 have died from cancers linked to radiation exposure.[19] **Figure 2-3** shows the power plant after the explosion, and **Figure 2-4** depicts the spread of radiation from the plant, as well as the areas that had to be controlled.

The public health community's immediate and long-term responsibility in response to the Chernobyl disaster was significant, including assessing the safety of the environment for human habitation, addressing the psychological impact of the disaster on affected populations, monitoring the long-term health and well-being of exposed populations, and planning for the treatment of untold numbers of current and future cancer patients.[19,20]

More recent, on March 11, 2011, a 9.0 magnitude earthquake and subsequent tsunami hit the east coast of Japan, causing widespread damage and loss of life, crippling the Fukushima Daiichi Nuclear Power Station. The full impact of this nuclear plant disaster is not yet fully known, but local populations had to be evacuated from their homes; radioactive iodine and cesium have been found in locally produced foods; and drinking water, seawater, soil, and air must be continually monitored.[21]

FIGURE 2-3 An Aerial View of Ukraine's Chernobyl Nucler Power Plant, Taken in May 1986, Several Days after the Explosion on April 26, 1986

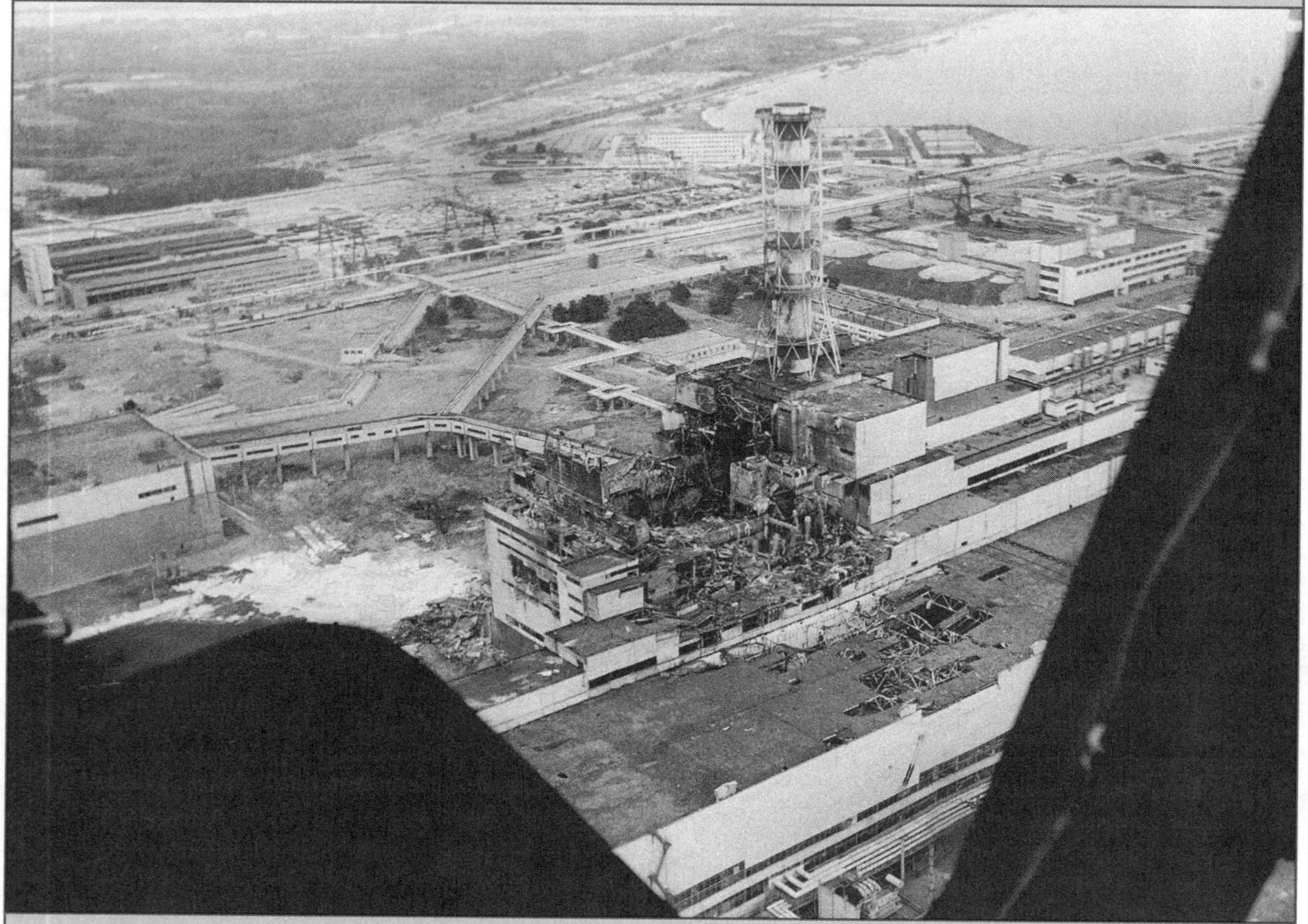

Source: © AP Photos.

FIGURE 2-4 Radiation Contamination after the Chernobyl Disaster

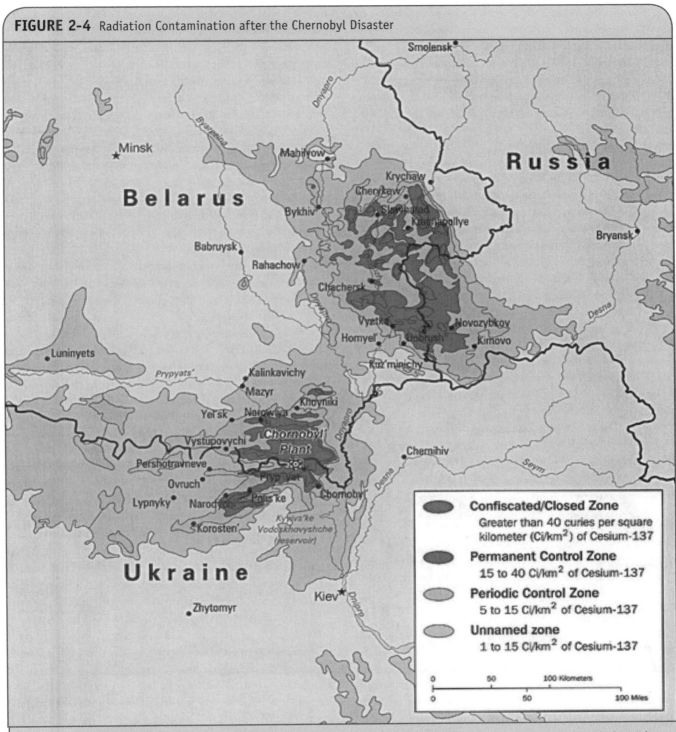

Legend:

Confiscated/Closed Zone
Greater than 40 curies per square kilometer (Ci/km^2) of Cesium-137

Permanent Control Zone
15 to 40 Ci/km^2 of Cesium-137

Periodic Control Zone
5 to 15 Ci/km^2 of Cesium-137

Unnamed zone
1 to 15 Ci/km^2 of Cesium-137

Source: Central Intelligence Agency. "Radiation Contamination after the Chernobyl Disaster," Making the History of 1989, Item #173, http://chnm.gmu.edu/1989/items/show/173 (accessed March 3, 2011, 9:30 a.m.).

In addition to the public health risk of accidental radiological exposure, the global community continues to be concerned about the intentional use of a nuclear or radiological device. In April 2010, President Barack Obama called the global community to a Nuclear Security Summit, where the nations of the world clearly acknowledged the threat of nuclear terrorism. President Obama delivered the following statement:

> Two decades after the end of the Cold War, we face a cruel irony of history—the risk of a nuclear confrontation between nations has gone down, but the risk of nuclear attack has gone up.
>
> Nuclear materials that could be sold or stolen and fashioned into a nuclear weapon exist in dozens of nations. Just the smallest amount of plutonium—about the size of an apple—could kill and injure hundreds of thousands of innocent people. Terrorist networks such as al Qaeda have tried to acquire the material for a nuclear weapon, and if they ever succeeded, they would surely use it. Were they to do so, it would be a catastrophe for the world—causing extraordinary loss of life, and striking a major blow to global peace and stability.
>
> In short, it is increasingly clear that the danger of nuclear terrorism is one of the greatest threats to global security—to our collective security.[22]

The International Atomic Energy Agency (IAEA) receives, on average, a report every 2 days on an incident of illicit trafficking of nuclear or radiological material.[23] Unfortunately, the nuclear and radiological threat is very real, and it is essential that the public health community be prepared.

BIOLOGICAL THREATS

The biological threat can be thought of as a continuum, including everything from naturally occurring diseases to the intentional release of a biological agent. This book will focus on the threat from natural disease and emerging and pandemic threats in later chapters; in this chapter, we focus exclusively on the intentional threat. *Biological warfare* (BW) is the military use of a biological agent to cause death or harm to humans, animals, or plants. In warfare, the targets of biological agents are typically governments, armed forces, or resources that might affect the ability of a nation to attack others or defend itself. Similarly, *bioterrorism* (BT) is the threat or use of a biological agent to harm or kill humans, plants, or animals. Unlike BW, though, the target of BT is typically the civilian population or resources that might affect the civilian economy, and the aggressor is often a nonstate actor. *Agroterrorism* refers to the knowing or malicious use of biological agents to affect the agricultural industry or food supply.[24]

As with chemical and radiological threats, there is a long history of the intentional use of biological agents. One example that is cited regularly comes from the 1346–1347 siege by Mongols of the city of Kaffa, now Feodosija, Ukraine. The Mongols reportedly catapulted corpses contaminated with plague over the walls of the city, causing an outbreak of *Yersinia pestis*.[25] Another history example comes from 1767 when British troops gave smallpox-infested blankets to Native Americans, causing a massive outbreak of smallpox among this unexposed population.

There was little use of biological weapons during World War I. In fact, the only reported use was by Germany, who used anthrax and glanders to infect Allied livestock.[26(p 513)] After WWI, however, the Japanese began a robust offensive biological weapons program, housed in what was called "Unit 731." This unit was based in Harbin, Manchuria, and conducted extensive research and experiments, often using prisoners of war as subjects. In 1940, the Japanese dropped rice and wheat mixed with plague-carrying fleas over China and Manchuria, leading to localized plague outbreaks. In 1942, the United States began its offensive biological weapons program. (See **Box 2-3**.)

Several additional high-profile biological weapons events occurred starting in the late 1970s. In 1979, in the Siberian town of Sverdlovsk in the Soviet Union (now Yekaterinburg), at least 77 people became ill with anthrax, resulting in 66 fatalities. Originally, the Soviet Union claimed that the cause of the outbreak was bad meat and the route of infection gastrointestinal. In reality, the cause of the outbreak was human error—someone forgot to replace a filter—at a military installation that was producing anthrax for offensive purposes. The anthrax escaped into the air, and those who became ill fell within the wind plume leading directly from the military compound, as depicted in **Figure 2-5**. In 1992, Boris Yeltsin admitted to the international community that the source of the anthrax in this outbreak came from the offensive military production site and not from consumption of infected meat.[27,28(p 163)]

Other events linked to the Soviet Union occurred during the same time period. Starting in 1976 in Laos, 1978 in Cambodia, and 1979 in Afghanistan, there were reports of chemical or toxin weapons use against the Hmong, Khmer, and Mujuhadin, respectively (see **Figure 2-6**). The alleged attacks were often said to begin with a helicopter or plane flying over

BOX 2-3 U.S. Offensive Biological Warfare Program, 1942–1972

1942 The National Academies of Sciences Biological Warfare Committee recommends that the United States should develop an offensive and defensive biological weapons program. Secretary of War Henry L. Stimson recommends to the president that a civilian organization be set up to run the program, and the president approves. The War Research Service (WRS) is established, and George Merck accepts the leadership position.

1943 A biological weapons research and development facility is constructed in Frederick, Maryland, at Camp Detrick, and becomes operational. Research begins on the offensive potential of botulinum toxin and anthrax.

1944 The biological warfare program is transferred from the WRS to the War Department. The War Department divides the program between the Chemical Warfare Service (CWS) and the U.S. Army Surgeon General. CWS works mostly on offensive research and production, while the Surgeon General focuses more on defensive measures. The research and development program is housed at Camp Detrick. An existing industrial plant near Terre Haute, Indiana, is acquired for conversion to a biological weapons production plant. Research on biological agents is expanded to include brucellosis, psittacosis, tularemia, and glanders.

1946 The War Department publicly acknowledges that the United States has developed an offensive biological weapons program.

1950 Several open-air sea tests are conducted using simulants. Field testing is also conducted at Dugway Proving Ground. The construction of a production facility at Pine Bluff Arsenal is authorized.

1950–1960 Research and production of at least seven biological agents continues. Airborne testing continues, and the program is expanded.

1960–1970 Funding for the biological warfare program starts to decline, but the army continues to work on antipersonnel, antiplant, and antianimal agents and runs several open-air tests using simulants in populated areas. The program also works on developing vaccines for defensive purposes.

1969 President Richard Nixon directs the National Security Council to review the chemical and biological weapons policy. The Senate Armed Services Committee votes to zero-out funding for the biological weapons program and prohibit additional open-air testing. On November 25, President Nixon renounces the development, production, stockpiling, and use of biological warfare agents. The Department of Defense is ordered to destroy existing biological weapons and engage in research only for defensive purposes.

1971–1973 The United States destroys all biological warfare agents and munitions.

1972 The United States signs the Biological and Toxin Weapons Convention.

1975 The Senate approves and the president ratifies both the Biological and Toxin Weapons Convention and the Geneva Protocol of 1925.

Sources: The Henry L. Stimson Center. History of the US Offensive Biological Warfare Program (1941–1973). *Biological and Chemical Weapons.* Available at: http://www.stimson.org/topics/biological-chemical-weapons/. Accessed July 10, 2010; and Smart JK. History of Chemical and Biological Warfare: An American Perspective. *Textbook of Military Medicine: Medical Aspects of Chemical and Biological Warfare.* Washington, DC: Office of the Surgeon General, US Department of the Army; 1989.

a village or resistance group and release of a colored gas that would fall in a manner that often looked, felt, and sounded like rain. The most common color reported was yellow, and thus the collective name for these incidents became "Yellow Rain." The alleged causative agent was trichothecene mycotoxin (T2), and the alleged supplier of this toxin was the Soviet Union, who provided it to the Pathet Lao in Laos, to the Vietnamese for use against Khmer resistance groups in Cambodia, and for direct use by the Soviets in Afghanistan. High levels of morbidity and mortality were associated with the allegations

FIGURE 2-5 Wind Plume from Military Installation Allegedly Producing Anthrax in Sverdlosk and the Location of Anthrax Cases in 1979

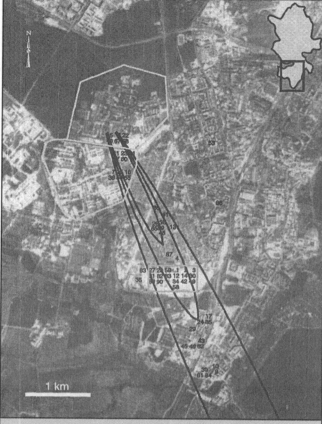

Source: Meselson, M.J., J. Guillemin, M. Hugh-Jones, et al. (1994), The Sverdlovsk Anthrax Outbreak of 1979, *Science*, 266, no. 5188:1202–1208.

difficult it is to distinguish between a naturally occurring event and an intentional release of an agent, which enables plausible deniability on the part of the perpetrators. Members of the Epidemic Intelligence Service (EIS) from the CDC were called in to help with the investigation. While the EIS officers felt that something was not right with the outbreak, they were unable to definitively say that the cases were not of natural origin. It was not until a year after the event, when a member of the cult confessed to authorities, that the public health officials were able to fully understand the nature of the outbreak.[31,32]

The most well-known bioterrorism event in the United States occurred in the fall of 2001, just weeks after the 9/11 attacks. The case, eventually named "Amerithrax" by the Federal Bureau of Investigation (FBI), involved finely milled anthrax sent through the mail, targeting senators and media outlets. **Figure 2-7** shows pictures of two of the anthrax letters, and **Figure 2-8** is the epidemic curve of the attacks and subsequent cases. In all, 22 people became ill and 5 died. Thousands of postal workers, congressional staff, and other potentially exposed individuals received prophylactic antibiotics and were offered vaccines. Thousands more were potentially exposed during this incident, and many more who were worried about possible effects of exposure demanded antibiotics from their personal physicians. Vast sums of money were spent decontaminating post office facilities and Senate office buildings. In 2010, the FBI finally closed the Amerithrax case, claiming the perpetrator was a U.S. government researcher at Fort Detrick, named Bruce Ivins. Dr. Ivins committed suicide before being formally charged and thus never stood trial.

The total disruption caused by what was—in the end—the equivalent of about a sugar packet amount of anthrax is impressive. The vast infrastructure and funding that came about in response to the attack was even more impressive. This will be discussed more fully in subsequent chapters.

Biological Agents

For a biological agent to be an effective weapon, it should ideally (from the perpetrator's perspective) have high toxicity; be fast acting; be predictable in its impact; have a capacity for survival outside the host for enough time to infect a victim; be relatively indestructible by air, water, or food purification; and be susceptible to medical countermeasures available to the attacker but not to the intended victim(s). Of the many biological agents that exist in nature (including parasites, fungi and yeasts, bacteria, rickettsia and Chlamydia, viruses, prions, and toxins), most effort is directed at a small group of bacteria, viruses, and toxins as the primary source of potential biological weapons. (See **Box 2-4**.)

of Yellow Rain. In 1982, the United States estimated that more than 10,700 people had been killed. Some estimated the loss of life to be much greater, particularly within the Hmong community. Some estimates go up to 20,000, and the Lao Human Rights Council puts the number as high as 40,000.[29,30]

The first large-scale bioterrorist event in the United States occurred in 1984 in The Dalles, Oregon. The Rajneeshee Cult, living in the area at the time, wished to influence a local election. Their plan was to make people in the town too sick to show up to vote in the election, have all of the members of the cult vote, and thereby vote their candidate into office. As a trial run, cult members infected multiple salad bars in local restaurants with salmonella. As a result, 751 people became ill, and 45 were hospitalized. This case demonstrates how

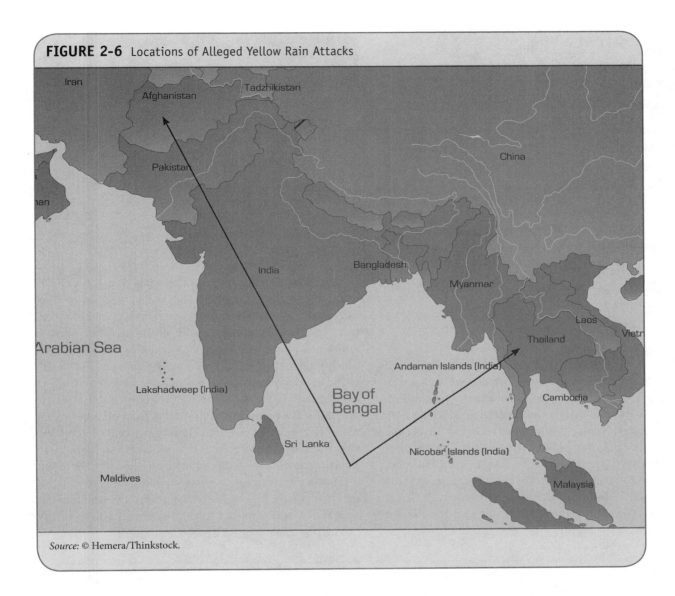

FIGURE 2-6 Locations of Alleged Yellow Rain Attacks

Source: © Hemera/Thinkstock.

Classification of Biological Agents

Two major characterizations are used to classify biological agents. The first, used more by policy planners at the federal level, looks at the spectrum of agents and defines them as:

- *Traditional:* Traditional agents are naturally occurring microorganisms or toxins that have long been connected with bioterrorism or biological warfare either because they have been used in the past or they have been studied for use. There are a finite number of agents that are relatively well understood. The policy and public health community has devised specific plans to address the potential use of these agents. Examples include smallpox and anthrax.

- *Enhanced:* Enhanced agents are traditional biological agents that have been altered to circumvent medical countermeasures. This group includes agents that are resistant to antibiotics.
- *Emerging:* This category includes any naturally occurring emerging organism or emerging infectious disease. Examples include severe acute respiratory syndrome (SARS), H5N1, and novel H1N1.
- *Advanced:* The final category on the spectrum of biological threats encompasses novel pathogens and other artificial agents that are engineered in laboratories. It is virtually impossible to plan for the specific threats posed by this category of agents, thus forcing policy makers to look at biological threats with a much broader strategic approach.

FIGURE 2-7 One of the Anthrax Letters Sent to Senator Leahy

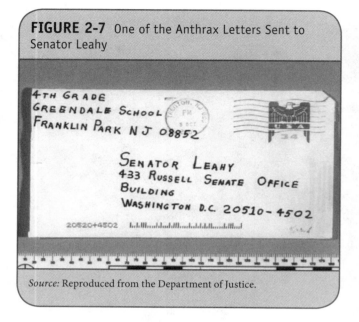

Source: Reproduced from the Department of Justice.

BOX 2-4 Biological Agents in Nature

Bacteria	Free-living unicellular organisms
Viruses	Core of DNA or RNA surrounded by a coat of protein; require host cell to replicate; much smaller than bacteria
Toxins	Toxic substances produced by living organisms

The second classification method for biological threat agents is the Category A, B, and C list, shown in **Box 2-5**. (Pictures of several agents from this list can be found in **Figures 2-9 to 2-14**.) This categorization originated with a 1999 CDC Strategic Planning Workgroup, which looked at the public health impacts of biological agents, the potential of those agents to be effective weapons, public perception, fear, and preparedness requirements. They also examined existing lists, including the Select Agent Rule list, the Australia Group list for export control, and the World Health Organization list of biological weapons.[33]

The resulting lists begin with Category A, which includes the highest-priority pathogens with the highest threat. They can cause large-scale morbidity and mortality and often require specific preparedness plans on the part of the public health community. Category B includes the second-highest threat group. Most of the agents in this category are waterborne or foodborne. These agents have often been intentionally used in the past or were part of offensive research programs. The morbidity and mortality from these agents are not as significant as from Category A agents, but still considerable, and they often require the public health community to enhance surveillance and diagnostic capacity. The last group is Category C, which encompasses emerging pathogens or agents that have become resistant to medical countermeasures. These agents may cause high morbidity and mortality and may be easily produced and transmitted.[34]

FIGURE 2-8 Number of Bioterrorism–Related Anthrax Cases, by Date of Onset and Work Location. District of Columbia (DC), Florida (FL), New Jersey (NJ), and New York City (NYC), September 16–October 25, 2001

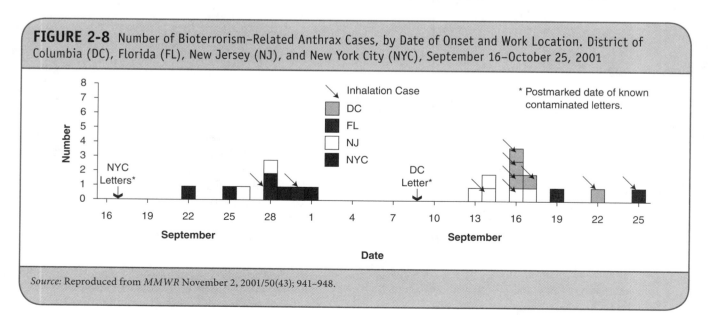

Source: Reproduced from *MMWR* November 2, 2001/50(43); 941–948.

BOX 2-5 Category A, B, and C Threat Agents

Category A
- *Bacillus anthracis* (anthrax)
- *Clostridium botulinum*
- *Yersinia pestis* (plague)
- Variola major (smallpox) and other pox viruses
- *Francisella tularensis* (tularemia)
- Viral hemorrhagic fevers
  - Arenaviruses
    - LCM, Junin virus, Machupo virus, Guanarito virus
    - Lassa Fever
  - Bunyaviruses
    - Hantaviruses
    - Rift Valley Fever
  - Flaviviruses
    - Dengue
  - Filoviruses
    - Ebola
    - Marburg

Category B
- *Burkholderia pseudomallei*
- *Coxiella burnetii* (Q fever)
- *Brucella* species (brucellosis)
- *Burkholderia mallei* (glanders)
- Ricin toxin (from *Ricinus communis*)
- Epsilon toxin of *Clostridium perfringens*
- Staphylococcus enterotoxin B
- Typhus fever (*Rickettsia prowazekii*)
- Food- and waterborne pathogens
  - Bacteria
    - Diarrheagenic *E. coli*
    - Pathogenic Vibrios
    - *Shigella* species
    - *Salmonella* species
  - *Listeria monocytogenes*
  - *Campylobacter jejuni*
  - *Yersinia enterocolitica*
- Viruses (Caliciviruses, Hepatitis A)
- Protozoa
  - *Cryptosporidium parvum*
  - *Cyclospora cayatanensis*
  - *Giardia lamblia*
  - *Entamoeba histolytica*
  - Toxoplasma
  - Microsporidia
- Additional viral encephalitides
  - West Nile Virus
  - LaCrosse
  - California encephalitis
  - Venezuelan equine encephalitis
  - Eastern equine encephalitis
  - Western equine encephalitis
  - Japanese Encephalitis Virus
  - Kyasanur Forest Virus

Category C
- Emerging infectious diseases (including Nipah)
- Tickborne hemorrhagic fever viruses
  - Crimean-Congo hemorrhagic fever virus
- Tickborne encephalitis viruses
- Yellow fever
- Multi-drug-resistant TB
- Influenza
- Other Rickettsias
- Rabies
- Severe acute respiratory syndrome–associated coronavirus (SARS-CoV)
- Antimicrobial resistance disease (excluding sexually transmitted diseases)

Source: Centers for Disease Control and Prevention. Bioterrorism Agents/Diseases—By Category. *Emergency Preparedness and Response.* Available at: http://www.bt.cdc.gov/agent/agentlist-category.asp. Accessed July 10, 2010.

Biological weapons are unique from other potential weapons of mass destruction in that the agents themselves are relatively available because many occur naturally and may be endemic in some parts of the world. The technology to work with these agents has progressed to a point where knowledge is widespread, and those with minimal formal education may possess the skills to work with and maliciously use certain agents. Compared with other weapons of mass destruction, biological weapons are inexpensive. While it is extraordinarily complicated to distribute biological weapons through a missile or other munition, other means of dissemination are quite easy (e.g., spraying salad bars). Intentional

FIGURE 2-9 Bacillus Anthracis

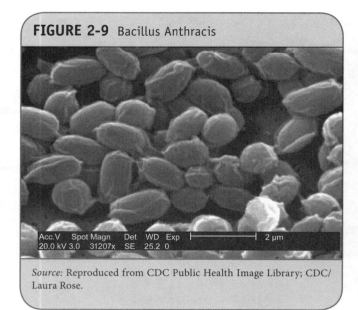

Source: Reproduced from CDC Public Health Image Library; CDC/ Laura Rose.

FIGURE 2-11 Salmonella

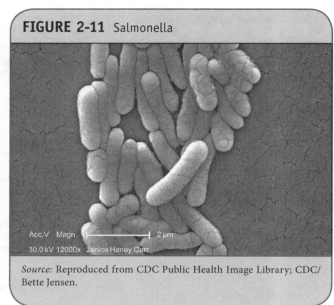

Source: Reproduced from CDC Public Health Image Library; CDC/ Bette Jensen.

FIGURE 2-10 Ebola Virus

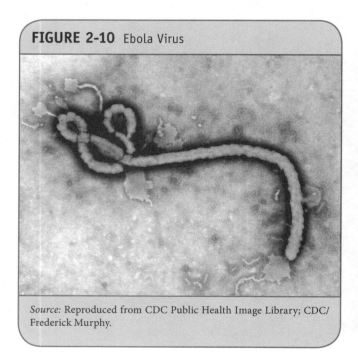

Source: Reproduced from CDC Public Health Image Library; CDC/ Frederick Murphy.

FIGURE 2-12 Giardia Protozoan

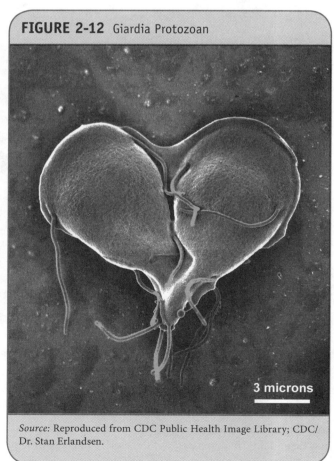

Source: Reproduced from CDC Public Health Image Library; CDC/ Dr. Stan Erlandsen.

FIGURE 2-13 West Nile Virus

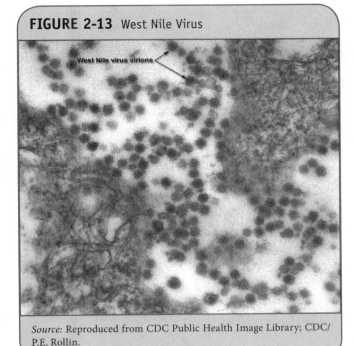

West Nile virus virions

Source: Reproduced from CDC Public Health Image Library; CDC/ P.E. Rollin.

attacks may be very difficult to detect and differentiate from a naturally occurring event, thus allowing for plausible deniability on the part of the offender.

Finally, biological weapons can be extremely lethal. A 1993 study by the now-defunct Congressional Office of Technology Assessment concluded that a crop duster plane flying over Washington, D.C., and disseminating 100 kg of anthrax powder had the potential to be more deadly than a 1-megaton hydrogen bomb. (See **Figure 2-15**.) An earlier study by the World Health Organization using a similar scenario of a line source dissemination of agent from an airplane also demonstrates the large-scale morbidity and mortality that can result from the intentional release of a biological weapon, as depicted in **Table 2-2**.

The Biological Threat

In December 2008, the Commission on the Prevention of Weapons of Mass Destruction Proliferation and Terrorism released the *World at Risk* report, in which they concluded there will likely be a biological attack some place in the world within the next 5 years, and biological weapons are to be considered a threat of primary importance to the United States.[35]

FIGURE 2-14 Influenza Virus

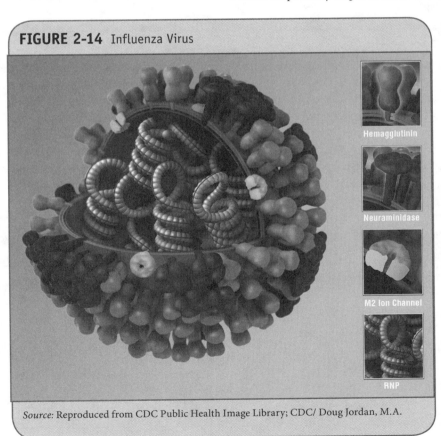

Hemagglutinin

Neuraminidase

M2 Ion Channel

RNP

Source: Reproduced from CDC Public Health Image Library; CDC/ Doug Jordan, M.A.

FIGURE 2-15 Lethality of Anthrax Compared to a Nuclear Weapon. 1993 Study by the Congressional Office of Technology Assessment

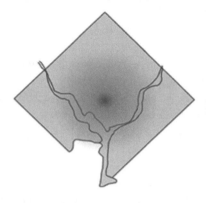

1 Megaton Hydrogen Bomb

Outline of Washington D.C.

570,000 -1,900,00 Deaths

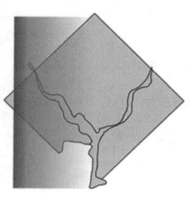

100 kg of Anthrax Powder

1,000,000 -3,000,00 Deaths

Source: U.S. Congress, Office of Technology Assessment, Proliferation of Weapons of Mass Destruction: Assessing the Risk, OTA-ISC-559 (Washington, DC: U.S. Government Printing Office, August 1993). Pages 53–54.

The threat of a biological weapons attack derives from multiple sources. An attack may be carried out by a lone actor, a terrorist group or an organization, or a state-sponsored program. At one point in time, there were probably a dozen nations that sponsored offensive biological weapons programs. Many fewer programs exist today,[36] but the agents created and knowledge gained from state-sponsored offensive programs have become threats unto themselves, as terrorist organizations lure scientists with financial incentives. For example, the former Soviet Union had an extensive offensive biological weapons program, spanning the military, KGB, and civilian sectors. In the civilian program, called Biopreparat, there were up to 40,000 scientists and technicians all working on biological weapons research and production.[37] This program was inherited by Russia after the fall of the Soviet Union, although in 1992 President Boris Yeltsin promised to

TABLE 2-2 Analysis of Morbidity and Mortality That Would Result from an Airplane Release of 50 kg of Agent Along a 2 km Line Upwind of a Population Center of 500,000

Agent	Downwind Reach (km)	Casualties	Dead
Rift Valley Fever	1	35,000	400
Tickborne enceph.	1	35,000	9,500
Typhus	5	85,000	19,000
Brucellosis	10	100,000	500
Q-fever	>20	125,000	150
Tularemia	>20	125,000	30,000
Anthrax	>>20	125,000	95,000

Source: Adapted from Health Aspects of Chemical and Biological Weapons, WHO, 1970.

FIGURE 2-16 Document Recovered from al Qaeda Facility at Tarnak Farms, Afghanistan

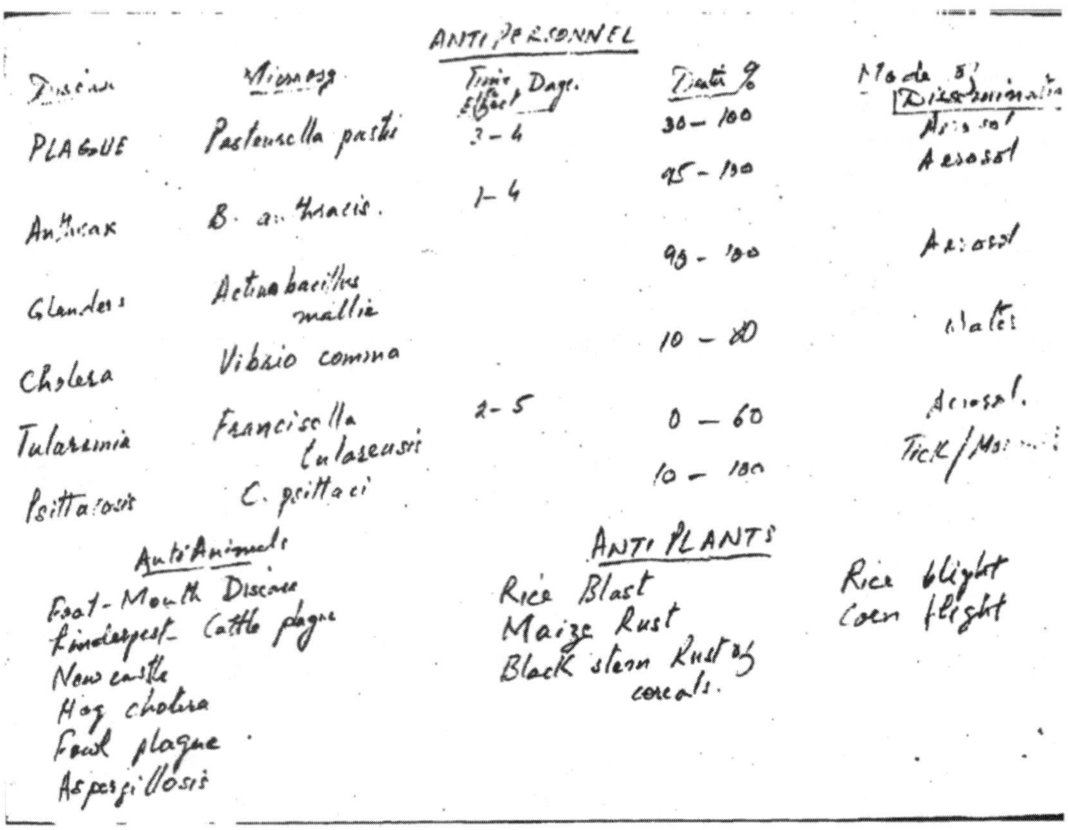

ANTI PERSONNEL

Disease	Microorg.	Time, Days, Effect	Death %	Mode of Dissemination
PLAGUE	Pasteurella pestis	3-4	30-100	Aerosol
Anthrax	B. anthracis.	1-4	95-100	Aerosol
Glanders	Actinobacillus mallie		93-100	Aerosol
Cholera	Vibrio comma		10-80	Water
Tularemia	Francisella tularensis	2-5	0-60	Aerosol.
Psittacosis	C. psittaci		10-100	Tick/Mo...

Anti Animals

Foot-Mouth Disease
Rinderpest Cattle plague
New castle
Hog cholera
Fowl plague
Aspergillosis

ANTI PLANTS

Rice Blast
Maize Rust
Black stem Rust of cereals.

Rice blight
Corn blight

Source: U.S. Department of Defense, Office of the Assistant Secretary of Defense (Public Affairs). Enduring Freedom Operational Update—Rear. Adm. Stufflebeem; Wednesday, October 31, 2001 - 1:30 p.m. EST.

terminate the program. While much effort and money have gone toward redirecting former weapons scientists into more peaceful lines of work (see description of cooperative threat reduction programs later in this book), it is unclear whether all of the scientists involved in the program or the materials they worked with are accounted for. Thus, the threat of knowledge and agents moving to other nations or terrorist organizations remains.

Terrorist organizations also present a significant threat that biological weapons will be used. As previously mentioned, the Rajneeshee cult successfully engaged in bioterrorism, as did Aum Shinrikyo. In addition to the sarin gas attack, Aum Shinrikyo had attempted to use biological weapons but was unsuccessful in causing any injuries (they used a vaccine strain of agent that would not cause disease and utilized inefficient dissemination mechanisms). When police raided their compound after the sarin attack, they found cultures of anthrax and botulism and spray tanks.[38]

Al Qaeda has yet to use biological weapons but has expressed interest in this means of terrorism. The United States found a facility in Afghanistan that had been used by al Qaeda, possibly to experiment with or eventually produce a biological weapon. At this location, called Tarnak Farms, several documents were found, including analyses of the potential casualties from different agents and notes about where to acquire seed cultures. (See **Figure 2-16**.) In addition to al Qaeda, at least 11 other terrorist organizations have expressed interest in using biological weapons.[39]

Overall, the current threat posed by biological weapons has increased significantly in the past decade. The potential consequences of an attack would go beyond population morbidity and mortality and could include such disruptions as a shutdown or slowdown of international travel and trade, economic shocks, potential civil disorder, public panic or confusion, and national or regional instability.

This text will examine the role of the public health community in addressing these threats and some of the challenges faced. Multiple sectors of society must work together to effectively prevent, prepare for, and manage the consequences of an attack, but the core of any effective detection and response capacity is public health. It is the public health community that can identify an event through population surveillance and clinical reporting. The public health community is central in mounting a response that treats those who are ill, protects those who may have been exposed, addresses immediate and long-term health consequences, and reconstitutes the infrastructure after the event has occurred.

KEY WORDS

Biological weapons
Bioterrorism
Chemical weapons
Radiological weapons
Toxins
Intentional use
Accidental exposures

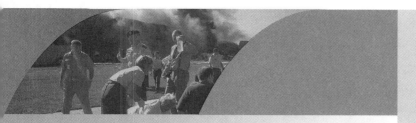

Discussion Questions

1. Do you agree with the *World at Risk* report that there will be a biological attack in the next 5 years? Why or why not?

2. What role would the public health community play if a radiological weapon was dispersed in a major metropolitan area?

3. Do you believe the public health community is aware of the threats from weapons of mass destruction? If not, what would you do to remedy the situation, and what information do you think would be important for public health professionals to know?

4. Do you believe the public health community is aware of or prepared for the potential for accidental chemical, biological or radiological exposure in its communities?

5. How should public health professionals communicate with security officials to be kept aware of the latest threats? Is that an appropriate role for public health?

REFERENCES

1. Chemical Weapons Convention. Available at: http://www.cwc.gov/cwc_treaty_full.html. Accessed June 26, 2010.

2. Nuclear Threat Initiative. Introduction to BW Terrorism. *BW Terrorism Tutorial*. 2004. Available at: http://www.nti.org/h_learnmore/bwtutorial/chapter01_03.html. Accessed June 26, 2010.

3. Hu H, Fine J, Epstein P, Kelsey K, Reynolds P, Walker B. Tear Gas—Harassing Agent or Toxic Chemical Weapon? *JAMA*. August 1989;262(5):660–663.

4. Fitzgerald GJ. Chemical Warfare and Medical Response During World War I. *American Journal of Public Health*. April 2008;98(4).

5. Chronology of Major Events in the History of Biological and Chemical Weapons. *James Martin Center for Nonproliferation Studies*. August 2008. Available at: http://cns.miis.edu/cbw/pastuse.htm. Accessed July 7, 2010.

6. Kang HK, Dalager NA, Needham LL, et al. Health Status of Army Chemical Corps Vietnam Veterans Who Sprayed Defoliant in Vietnam. *American Journal of Industrial Medicine*. November 2006;49(11):875–884.

7. Stellman JM, Stellman SD, Christian R, Weber T, Tomasallo C. The extent and patterns of usage of Agent Orange and other herbicides in Vietnam. *Nature*. April 2003;22:681–687.

8. Mossiker F. *The affair of the poisons: Louis XIV, Madame de Montespan, and one of history's great unsolved mysteries*, 1st ed. Knopf; 1969.

9. Vale A. What lessons can we learn from the Japanese sarin attacks? *Przegląd lekarski*. 2005;62(6):528–532.

10. World Health Organization. *The World Health Report 2007: A Safer Future—Global Public Health Security in the 21st Century*. 2007.

11. UN News Centre. Toxic wastes caused deaths, illnesses in Côte d'Ivoire—UN expert. *United Nations*. September 16, 2009. Available at: http://www.un.org/apps/news/story.asp?NewsID=32072. Accessed July 8, 2010.

12. Polgreen L, Simons M. Global Sludge Ends in Tragedy for Ivory Coast. *The New York Times*. October 2, 2006. Available at: http://www.nytimes.com/2006/10/02/world/africa/02ivory.html. Accessed July 8, 2010.

13. Agence France-Presse. Poison gas sweeps Nigerian city, 300 sickened. *Google News*. May 30, 2010. Available at: http://www.google.com/hostednews/afp/article/ALeqM5jZtgv1xTH1e4KIGRTu38lLtrdCEA. Accessed July 8, 2010.

14. Sharma DC. Bhopal: 20 years on. *The Lancet*. January 2005;365(9454):111–112.

15. Durham B. The Background and History of Manmade Disasters. *Topics in Emergency Medicine*. June 2002;24(2):1–14.

16. Centers for Disease Control and Prevention. Acute Radiation Syndrome (ARS): A Fact Sheet for the Public. *Emergency Preparedness and Response*. May 10, 2006. Available at: http://www.bt.cdc.gov/radiation/ars.asp. Accessed July 8, 2010.

17. Centers for Disease Control and Prevention. Radiation Emergencies—Information for Public Health Professionals. *Emergency Preparedness and Response*. March 31, 2010. Available at: http://www.bt.cdc.gov/radiation/publichealth.asp. Accessed July 8, 2010.

18. International Atomic Energy Agency. The Radiological Accident in Goiânia. 1988. Available at: http://www-pub.iaea.org/MTCD/publications/PDF/Pub815_web.pdf. Accessed July 8, 2010.

19. The Chernobyl Forum: 2003–2005. *Chernobyl's Legacy: Health, Environmental and Socio-Economic Impacts and Recommendations to the Governments of Belarus, the Russian Federation and Ukraine*. International Atomic Energy Agency (IAEA). April 2006. Available at: http://www.iaea.org/Publications/Booklets/Chernobyl/chernobyl.pdf. Accessed July 8, 2010.

20. Jargin SV. Overestimation of Thyroid Cancer Incidence after the Chernobyl Accident. *BMJ*. October 11, 2008. Available at: http://www.bmj.com/cgi/eletters/316/7136/952#202977. Accessed July 8, 2010.

21. World Health Organization, Western Pacific Region Japan earthquake and tsunami. Situation Report No. 33, 11 May 2011. Available at: http://www.wpro.who.int/NR/rdonlyres/B614B476-46F1-4094-846D-F5B-9D5BD0FB7/0/Sitrep3311May.pdf. Accessed May 18, 2011.

22. The White House, Office of the Press Secretary. Remarks by the President at the Opening Plenary Session of the Nuclear Security Summit. April 13, 2010. Available at: http://www.whitehouse.gov/the-press-office/remarks-president-opening-plenary-session-nuclear-security-summit. Accessed July 8, 2010.

23. International Atomic Energy Agency (IAEA). Statement at Nuclear Security Summit by IAEA Director General Yukiya Amano. *Statements of the Director General*. April 13, 2010. Available at: http://www.iaea.org/NewsCenter/Statements/2010/amsp2010n007.html. Accessed July 8, 2010.

24. Monke J. CRS Report for Congress: Agroterrorism: Threats. *Federation of American Scientists*. August 13, 2004. Available at: http://www.fas.org/irp/crs/RL32521.pdf. Accessed July 10, 2010.

25. Wheelis M. Biological Warfare at the 1346 Siege of Caffa. *Emerging Infectious Diseases*. September 2002;8(9):971–975.

26. Lesho ME, Dorsey MD, Bunner CD. Feces, Dead Horses, and Fleas—Evolution of the Hostile Use of Biological Agents. *Western Journal of Medicine*. June 1998;168(6):512–516.

27. Meselson M., Guillemin J, Hugh-Jones et al. The Sverdlovsk anthrax outbreak of 1979. *Science*. November 1994;266(5188):1202–1208.

28. Guillemin J. *Anthrax: The Investigation of a Deadly Outbreak*. University of California Press; 2001.

29. Katz R. *Yellow Rain Revisited: Lessons Learned for the Investigation of Chemical and Biological Weapons Allegations*. Dissertation ed. Princeton, NJ: Princeton University; 2005.

30. Katz R, Singer B. Can an attribution assessment be made for Yellow Rain? *Politics and the Life Sciences*. 2007;26(1):24–42.

31. Török TJ, Tauxe RV, Wise RP, et al. A large community outbreak of Salmonellosis caused by intentional contamination of restaurant salad bars. *JAMA*. August 1997;278(5):389–385.

32. Carus WS. The Rajneeshees (1984). In: Tucker JB, ed. *Toxic Terror: Assessing Terrorist Use of Chemical and Biological Weapons*. Cambridge, MA: MIT Press; 2000.

33. Elrod S. Category A–C agents. In: Katz R, Zilinikas R, eds. *Encyclopedia of Bioterrorism Defense*, 2nd ed. Wiley and Sons; May 2011.

34. Centers for Disease Control and Prevention. Bioterrorism Agents/Diseases—By Category. *Emergency Preparedness and Response*. Available at: http://www.bt.cdc.gov/agent/agentlist-category.asp. Accessed July 10, 2010.

35. Graham B, Talent J, Allison G, et al. *World at Risk: The Report of the Commission on the Prevention of WMD Proliferation and Terrorism*. December 2008. Available at: http://www.preventwmd.org/report/worldatrisk_full.pdf. Accessed July 10, 2010.

36. U.S. Department of State. *Adherence to and Compliance with Arms Control, Nonproliferation, and Disarmament Agreements and Commitments*. August 2005. Available at: http://www.state.gov/documents/organization/52113.pdf. Accessed July 10, 2010.

37. Alibek K. *Biohazard: The Chilling True Story of the Largest Covert Biological Weapons Program in the World—Told from Inside by the Man Who Ran It*. New York: Dell Publishing; 1999.

38. Clinehens MNA. *Aum Shinrikyo and Weapons of Mass Destruction: A Case Study*. Air Command and Staff College, Air University. April 2000. Available at: http://www.au.af.mil/au/awc/awcgate/acsc/00-040.pdf. Accessed July 10, 2010.

39. U.S. Department of State, Office of the Coordinator for Counterterrorism. *Country Reports on Terrorism 2009*. U.S. Department of State. August 2010. Available at: http://www.state.gov/documents/organization/141114.pdf. Accessed November 19, 2010.

Threats from Naturally Occurring Disease

INTRODUCTION

This chapter describes the links between disease and security and explores how and why naturally occurring disease events can and sometimes do become national security threats. We define key terms, explore the historical evolution of the policy commitments to disease as a security threat, and review several recent examples of disease outbreaks that have forced the once separate public health and security communities to reexamine how we view naturally occurring disease outbreaks in the context of security and preparedness.

Before beginning our discussion, we must first define the term *health security*. There has been much discussion in recent years about the "securitization of health," with some individuals even addressing the "healthification of security."[1] While several entities have attempted to define this term,[2,3,4,5] no consensus has been reached around what exactly health security means.

The definition of health security in **Box 3-1** is provided by the U.S. National Health Security Strategy, which empha-sizes a continual state of preparedness necessary to protect and respond to health threats. More specific, the National Health Security Strategy explains that a health emergency, such as a large outbreak of a naturally occurring infectious disease, can affect the workforce; the ability to provide food, water, and services; and economic productivity—all of which can destabilize society and governments.[3(p 3)]

The World Health Organization (WHO), on the other hand, defines health security as the activities that are necessary to "minimize vulnerability to acute public health events that endanger the collective health of populations." The WHO also adds that health security can affect "economic or political stability, trade, tourism, access to goods and services, and . . . demographic stability."[5(p ix)]

Each of these definitions embraces the notion that the health of a population—which can be affected by human behavior, disease, and natural and man-made threats—directly affects the security of a nation. Thus, a multisector approach is needed to effectively address health security. The security community must fully understand the capacity of the public health sector to prepare for, respond to, and recover from a health emergency. As stated by the director general of the WHO, public health security is both a "collective aspiration and a mutual responsibility."[5(p vii)]

EVOLUTION OF DISEASE AND SECURITY LINKS

Massive disease outbreaks, such as the 1918 influenza pandemic that touched every sector of society and killed millions around the world,[6] clearly affected the security and prosperity of populations. Yet, the formal recognition of disease as a security threat did not begin to take form until the 1990s. Fueled by the HIV/AIDS pandemic, emergence of Ebola, re-emergence of cholera, introduction of new subtypes of dengue in the Americas, and the onset of drug-resistant tuberculosis (TB), the Clinton administration issued an assessment in 1996: Addressing the Threat of Emerging Infectious Diseases.[7] The Presidential Decision Directive called for strengthening the national infectious disease surveillance system, building a global surveillance and response system, and expanding the mandate of the Department of Defense to "better protect American citizens."[8]

In 2000, greater political recognition of the link between health and security was initiated. In January, the National Intelligence Council (a think tank for the U.S. intelligence community) released a report, titled "The Global Infectious Disease Threat and Its Implications for the United States." This report responded to concerns by U.S. government officials that the spread of infectious diseases may affect health, economics, and national security. The report signaled the intelligence community's interest in considering disease as a nontraditional threat to national security.[9]

Also, in January 2000, the UN Security Council recognized the HIV/AIDS pandemic as a security issue.[10] This marked the first time the Security Council considered an infectious disease as a threat to security. Several months later, on April 29, 2000, the Clinton administration formally recognized infectious diseases as a threat to U.S. national security.[11] Together, these actions marked a paradigm shift in thinking about security threats and the relationship between disease and security. In theory, these events should have led to increased funding, political support, and actions to ad-

FIGURE 3-1 National Security Strategy, 2002

THE NATIONAL SECURITY STRATEGY OF THE UNITED STATES OF AMERICA

SEPTEMBER 2002

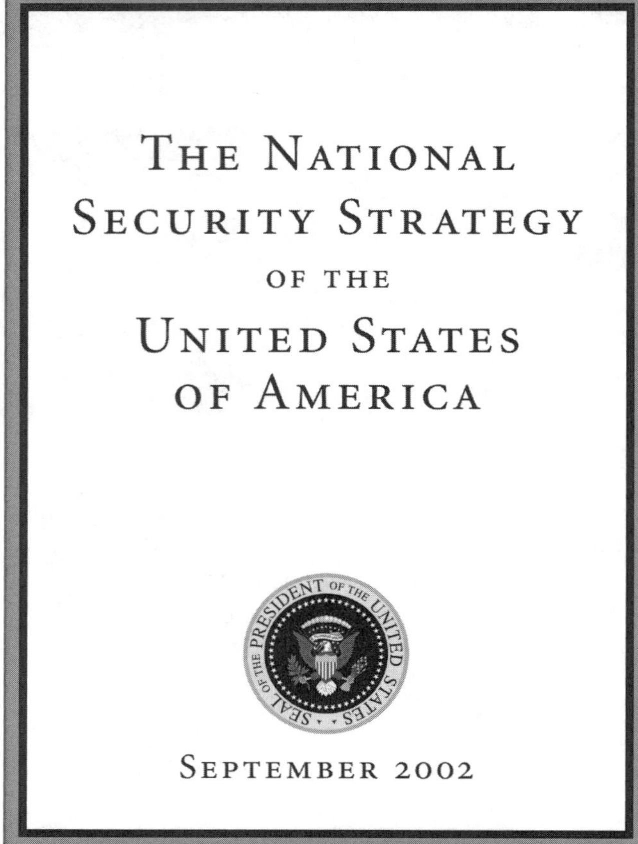

Source: Reproduced from National Security Strategy, 2002.

dress the interplay between health and security. In reality, however, it has taken almost a decade to solidify health as a security threat and to attract the attention and resources of the security community.

The evolution of the understanding and commitment to disease as a nontraditional security threat by senior security officials in the U.S. government can be seen in the series of National Security Strategies published over the course of a decade. (See **Figures 3-1, 3-2, and 3-3**.) In 2002, President George W. Bush released the National Security Strategy, which was heavily influenced by the terrorist attacks of September 11, 2001 and the anthrax letters immediately afterward. Public health and health promotion are mentioned several times but only as components of development assistance. HIV/AIDS is mentioned as a condition that, due to its devastation to sub-Saharan Africa, requires direct assistance. And medical preparedness for bioterror threats is mentioned briefly, in the

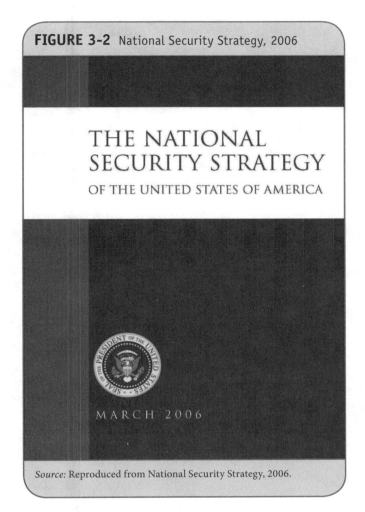

FIGURE 3-2 National Security Strategy, 2006

Source: Reproduced from National Security Strategy, 2006.

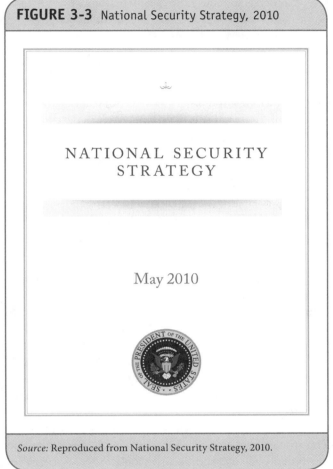

FIGURE 3-3 National Security Strategy, 2010

Source: Reproduced from National Security Strategy, 2010.

sense that preparedness efforts will also benefit infectious disease and other mass-casualty events.[12] Both public health preparedness and disease are addressed in the strategy, but no direct link is made between disease and security.

In 2006, President Bush released an updated National Security Strategy that focused slightly more on the threat of both biological weapons and infectious diseases. The updated strategy explicitly mentions the need to improve capacity to detect and respond to biological attacks, as well as the need to secure dangerous pathogens, strengthen global surveillance, develop medical countermeasures, and improve public health infrastructure—all in support of countering a biological attack. In regard to disease, the strategy declares that pandemics pose "a catastrophic challenge to national security with risks to social disorder."[13] At the time, the country was preparing for a potential pandemic of H5N1 and had become very aware of the potential threat posed by this strain of influenza. In addition to declaring the need to prepare for the pandemic

threat, the strategy also calls for transparent public health systems and emphasizes the need for governmental efforts to control and contain HIV/AIDS, TB, and malaria.

The evolution of health as a security threat culminates at the end of the decade with the Obama administration's introduction of the 2010 National Security Strategy.[14] For the first time, the political administration fully recognized the relationship between health and security, as well as the need to strengthen public health systems to address the biological threat. To counter the biological threat, the strategy provides the following guidance:

> The effective dissemination of a lethal biological agent within a population center would endanger the lives of hundreds of thousands of people and have unprecedented economic, societal, and political consequences. We must continue to work at home with first responders and health

officials to reduce the risk associated with unintentional or deliberate outbreaks of infectious disease and to strengthen our resilience across the spectrum of high-consequence biological threats. We will work with domestic and international partners to protect against biological threats by promoting global health security and reinforcing norms of safe and responsible conduct; obtaining timely and accurate insight on current and emerging risks; taking reasonable steps to reduce the potential for exploitation; expanding our capability to prevent, attribute, and apprehend those who carry out attacks; communicating effectively with all stakeholders; and helping to transform the international dialogue on biological threats.[14(p 24)]

In addition to addressing the biological threat, the 2010 strategy fully and explicitly defines the connections between pandemic and infectious diseases and security, and the need to build and maintain public health infrastructure to protect population health *and* national security, as seen in **Box 3-2**.

In December 2009, the Obama administration released the first ever National Health Security Strategy.[3] The purpose of the strategy, mandated by the Pandemic and All Hazards Preparedness Act of 2006 (PAHPA), was to provide a common vision for how the United States would achieve health security. This strategy, which we looked at earlier in the chapter regarding its definition of health security, looks at health security as a state that can be achieved through public health preparedness, community resilience, integrated response teams, and overall planning.

DEFINING THE LINK BETWEEN DISEASE AND SECURITY

We have traced the political evolution of health security, but how exactly does health affect national security? There are both direct and indirect links between health and national security, discussed in **Box 3-3**.

The direct impact of disease on national security arises from the potential proliferation or use of a biological weapon, or the intentional spread of disease within specific populations. In addition, the impact of disease on the armed forces directly affects security because morbidity and mortality affect "readiness"—the ability of the nation to defend itself militarily and to engage in armed battles around the world. It is interesting to note that until World War II, more soldiers died from infectious diseases than from direct combat injuries.[15] Disease altered the outcomes of conflicts and affected

---

BOX 3-2 May 2010 National Security Strategy: Section on Pandemic and Infectious Disease

The threat of contagious disease transcends political boundaries, and the ability to prevent, quickly detect, and contain outbreaks with pandemic potential has never been so important. An epidemic that begins in a single community can quickly evolve into a multinational health crisis that causes millions to suffer, as well as spark major disruptions to travel and trade. Addressing these transnational risks requires advance preparation, extensive collaboration with the global community, and the development of a resilient population at home.

Recognizing that the health of the world's population has never been more interdependent, we are improving our public health and medical capabilities on the front lines, including domestic and international disease surveillance, situational awareness, rapid and reliable development of medical countermeasures to respond to public health threats, preparedness education and training, and surge capacity of the domestic health care system to respond to an influx of patients due to a disaster or emergency. These capabilities include our ability to work with international partners to mitigate and contain disease when necessary.

We are enhancing international collaboration and strengthening multilateral institutions in order to improve global surveillance and early warning capabilities and quickly enact control and containment measures against the next pandemic threat. We continue to improve our understanding of emerging diseases and help develop environments that are less conducive to epidemic emergence. We depend on U.S. overseas laboratories, relationships with host nation governments, and the willingness of states to share health data with nongovernmental and international organizations. In this regard, we need to continue to work to overcome the lack of openness and a general reluctance to share health information. Finally, we seek to mitigate other problem areas, including limited global vaccine production capacity, and the threat of emergent and reemergent disease in poorly governed states.

Source: The White House. *The National Security Strategy*, pp. 48–49. May 2010. Available at: www.whitehouse.gov/sites/default/files/rss_viewer/national_security_strategy.pdf. Accessed July 25, 2010.

BOX 3-3 Strategic Implications of Global Health

The National Intelligence Council released a report in 2008 on the Strategic Implications of Global Health. This box, quoting text from the report, highlights the direct and indirect relationship between infectious diseases and U.S. national security.

- [A] number of infectious *and* non-infectious health conditions shape the world we live in—and by extension can impact U.S. interests. Infectious diseases for the foreseeable future, however, will remain the top health-related threat to U.S. national security:

- Americans at home will continue to be vulnerable to emerging and re-emerging infectious diseases—many of which will originate overseas (e.g., HIV/AIDS, West Nile, and dengue fever)—including a potential influenza pandemic or an outbreak of a "mystery" disease (e.g., SARS).

- Infectious diseases are likely to continue to significantly impact military operations. Particularly with deployments of U.S. military personnel to developing countries on the rise, U.S. forces could be increasingly vulnerable to mission-compromising outbreaks of diseases borne by insects or local food and water.

- In the case of multinational missions, health of U.S. forces—not to mention mission readiness—could be compromised by failure of coalition partners to provide adequate health protection measures to their troops.

- Infectious diseases *in concert with non-infectious conditions* are likely to slow socioeconomic development in developing and formerly communist countries of interest to the United States—with possible impacts on democratization and regime stability.

- Infectious disease-related embargoes and restrictions on travel and immigration—especially in the wake of an influenza pandemic—could cause diplomatic frictions between the United States and other countries.

- ... the possibility of a bioterrorist attack against U.S. civilian and military personnel overseas or in the United States could grow as more states and groups develop a biological warfare capability.

Source: National Intelligence Council. *Strategic Implications of Global Health.* December 2008. Available at: http://www.dni.gov/nic/PDF_GIF_otherprod/ICA_Global_Health_2008.pdf. Accessed July 25, 2010.

the balance of power among states. Even today, troop exposure to diseases affects morbidity and mortality and readiness. Hospital admissions from disease continue to outnumber injuries and wounds. (See **Figure 3-4**.) As a result, the military has invested significant resources in infectious disease research, building diagnostic laboratory capacity around the world, disease surveillance infrastructure, and vaccine development.[16,17,18,19]

Indirectly, disease affects security because it can create large-scale morbidity and mortality, leading to massive loss of life and affecting all sectors of society. Such morbidity and mortality could result in economic loss and even long-term deterioration of economic viability. Fear of disease, in addition to disease itself, can lead to societal disruption, which can lead to civil disorder, political unrest, and, ultimately, destabilization. Also, chronic diseases, now the leading cause of morbidity and mortality around the world, can indirectly affect economies, government stability, and military readiness in strategic countries and regions.[20]

The burden of infectious diseases, and emerging infectious diseases in particular, tends to affect regions and countries least able to address the threat.[5] The World Health

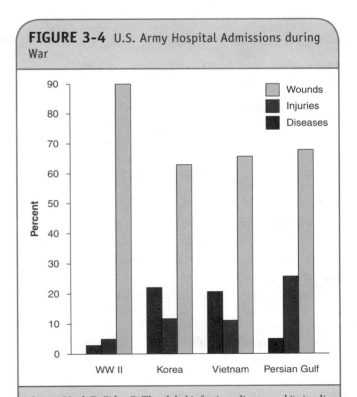

FIGURE 3-4 U.S. Army Hospital Admissions during War

Source: Noah D, Fidas G. The global infectious disease and its implications for the United States. Washington DC, National Intelligence Council (NIC), 2000. NIE 99-17D.

Organization, analyzing verified events of potential international public health concern between September 2003 and September 2006, found that the vast majority of events occurred in Africa (288). The western Pacific region was the second most affected with 108 events, followed by the eastern Mediterranean (89), Southeast Asia (81), Europe (78), and, finally, the Americas (41).[5](p 63) The regions where public health emergencies are most likely to emerge are the same regions experiencing critical shortages of healthcare personnel, and these regions tend to have the least developed healthcare infrastructure.[5,21] On top of this, many of the current and developing megacities (10 million people or more) can be found in the same regions as poor healthcare infrastructure, understaffed healthcare workforce, and the most public health emergencies.[21] This means that it is most probable that a public health emergency will emerge in a place that is under-staffed, under-resourced, and overpopulated—all conditions that may contribute to the spread of disease. And, given the speed and quantity of people and goods that move around the world, it is very possible for diseases to emerge in one part of the world and spread rapidly to all other populations. As President Obama explained in May 2009, "An outbreak in Indonesia can reach Indiana within days, and public health crises abroad can cause widespread suffering, conflict, and economic contraction."[22]

GLOBAL INTERCONNECTEDNESS AND THE SPREAD OF DISEASE

There have been several examples in recent history that underscore just how connected the world is and that people, animals, and pathogens travel the world with remarkable speed. Here are three examples of disease spreading around the world, reaching new populations and regions.

Monkeypox

In April 2003, a shipment of 800 small animals from Ghana arrived in Texas. Included in this shipment were Gambian rats, which were infected with monkeypox. The Gambian rats were kept in a location close enough to a group of prairie dogs to infect them with the disease. An Illinois animal vendor then sold these infected prairie dogs. Prairie dog owners—many of whom were children—were bitten by or touched either blood or rash on the infected animals (see **Figure 3-5**). This resulted in 71 cases of monkeypox throughout the midwestern United States (see **Table 3-1**).[23] Given that poxviruses, with the exception of chickenpox, are not commonly seen in the United States, the public health community was not prepared to treat the almost 80 cases and address public fear associated with the outbreak. In one instance, a 10-year-old girl struggled to

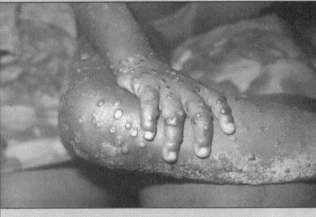

FIGURE 3-5 A Close-Up of Monkeypox Lesions on the Arm and Leg of a Female Child in Liberia

Source: Reproduced from CDC Public Health Image Library.

find a doctor who would treat her. When she did find medical care, she was relegated to a small medical staff willing to interact with her.[24]

Severe Acute Respiratory Syndrome

The best example of global interdependence, speed of air travel, and rapid movement of people comes from the SARS outbreak in 2003. The first case of what came to be called severe acute respiratory syndrome (SARS) emerged in November 2002 in Guangdong Province in southern China from exposure, slaughter, and consumption of small wild mam-

TABLE 3-1 Location and Number of Monkeypox Cases Resulting from 2003 Shipment of Infected Gambian Rats to the United States

STATE	# of cases
Illinois	12
Indiana	16
Kansas	1
Missouri	2
Ohio	1
Wisconsin	39
Total	**71**

Source: Centers for Disease Control and Prevention. Update: Multistate Outbreak of Monkeypox—Illinois, Indiana, Kansas, Missouri, Ohio, and Wisconsin, 2003. *Morbidity and Mortality Weekly Report.* July 2003;52(27):642–646.

mals. The outbreak grew over the course of several months, but the causative agent was not correctly identified, and little was done to contain the spread of disease. By early February 2003, there were almost 300 cases in Guangdong Province and five deaths.[25](p 6) China, however, did not report this emerging infectious disease to the outside world. The WHO queried China after receiving news of an outbreak through electronic reporting systems but was told it was a non-urgent acute respiratory syndrome.[25]

The worldwide spread of SARS began on February 21, 2003, as illustrated in **Figure 3-6**. An infected physician traveled to Hong Kong and stayed at the Metropole Hotel, where

FIGURE 3-6 How SARS Spread Around the World: Chain of Transmission among Guests at a Hotel in Hong Kong, 2003

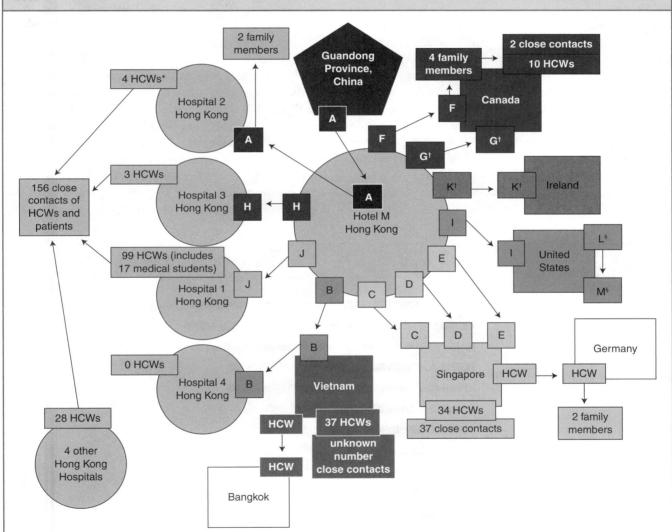

* Healthcare workers.
† All guests except G and K stayed on the 9th floor of the hotel. Guest G stayed on the 14th floor, and Guest K stayed on the 11th floor.
§ Guests L and M (spouses) were not at the Hotel M during the same time as index Guest A but were at the hotel during the same times as Guests G, H, and I, who were ill during this period.

Source: Morbidity and Mortality Weekly Report. March 28, 2003; 52(12).

he infected 12 other people at the hotel, who then left Hong Kong and brought the disease to the United States, Canada, Singapore, Vietnam, and Ireland.[26] In each instance, except in Ireland, these infected travelers then spread the disease in the next country. In at least one documented instance, SARS was spread on a transnational flight.[27] By September 2003, there had been 8,098 cases and 774 deaths reported in 29 countries.

The global experience with SARS and the actions taken to try to contain the disease as it spread throughout the world highlight our interconnectedness, as well as the challenges of global health governance. The WHO advised airlines to screen passengers and advised travelers to avoid all but essential travel to certain areas, resulting in significant economic consequences. Thailand saw a 55% decline in tourism, and SARS cut gross domestic product (GDP) growth in Vietnam by 1.1% in 2003. The full economic cost of the outbreak has been estimated to be approximately $30 to $50 billion, hitting Southeast Asia and Canada hardest.[25(p 91–136)] The epidemic led to discrimination, unnecessary isolation and quarantine, and political upheavals.[25(pp 91–136),28] SARS was a naturally occurring disease that caused morbidity and mortality, invoked fear, affected travel, led to population discrimination,

created an economic burden on certain nations, and affected security.

HIV/AIDS

The HIV/AIDS pandemic provides the most illustrative example to date of the ways in which a disease with high levels of morbidity and mortality can affect the security and viability of nations. HIV/AIDS has already caused approximately 25 million deaths worldwide.[29(p 31)] There were an estimated 33 million people living with HIV in 2007.[29(p 31)] Of all people living with HIV, 67% were in sub-Saharan Africa.[29(p 30)] The disease tends to affect the working-age population and has dramatically reduced life expectancy in some nations, in certain cases by more than 20 years.[29(p 13)] The disease has affected all sectors of society, from education to agriculture. The labor force in some countries has shrunk dramatically (see **Figure 3-7**), and the number of orphans from HIV/AIDS has grown—there are now nearly 12 million HIV/AIDS orphans in sub-Saharan Africa (see **Figure 3-8**). In Zimbabwe, almost a quarter of all children have lost at least one parent to HIV/AIDS.[29(p 163)] Without enough workers to sustain an economically viable society and with too few teachers and a growing number of orphans and children who cannot be

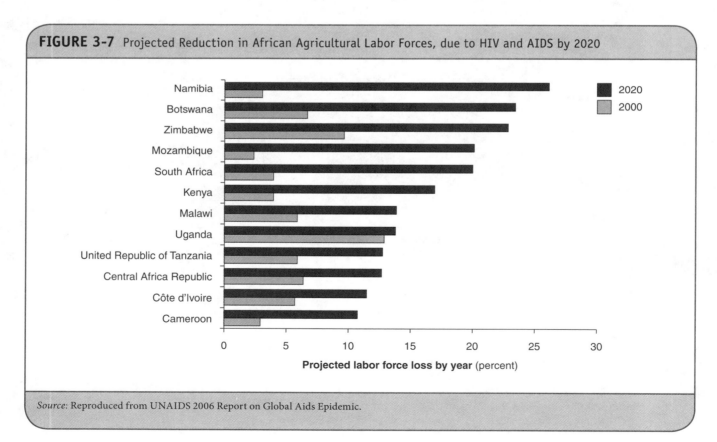

FIGURE 3-7 Projected Reduction in African Agricultural Labor Forces, due to HIV and AIDS by 2020

Source: Reproduced from UNAIDS 2006 Report on Global Aids Epidemic.

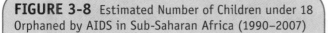

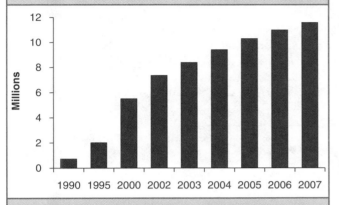

FIGURE 3-8 Estimated Number of Children under 18 Orphaned by AIDS in Sub-Saharan Africa (1990–2007)

Source: Reproduced from UNAIDS 2008 Report on Global Aids Epidemic.

provided for, nations without global support become almost destined for civil unrest and government instability. This point is emphasized in **Box 3-4**.

One of the most direct ways HIV/AIDS has affected national security is through the impact of the disease on militaries. Initial research suggested that armed conflict increased the spread and severity of HIV/AIDS in society. These claims, however, have not been proven through empirical analysis; more recent concern focuses on how disease may spread at the end of conflict.[30] The absolute numbers of HIV-positive

individuals in militaries, however, remain of great concern. Nations need to be capable of fielding healthy armed forces and, when the prevalence of disease among military-age citizens is high, this can be a challenge. For example, the prevalence of HIV has risen dramatically among Russian military recruits (see **Table 3-2**), posing unique challenges to both the civilian and military sectors to address the problem. As HIV/AIDS incidence and prevalence rise in countries such, as China and India, and because it retains its foothold in sub-Saharan Africa and Russia, the security implications of the disease cannot be underestimated.

RESPONSE

To date, the response to the health security nexus has been to try to establish stronger public health infrastructure and to direct assistance to address, contain, and mitigate natural disease threats. This has been accomplished by trying to strengthen global disease surveillance (see later chapters) and through disease and development assistance, primarily through the U.S. Global Health Initiative, the President's Emergency Plan for AIDS Relief (PEPFAR), the President's Malaria Initiative, and through the work of individual agencies providing assistance abroad, including the U.S. Agency for International Development (USAID), CDC, and the Department of Defense.

BOX 3-4 HIV/AIDS and Security: UN Security Council Resolution 1308 (17 July 2000)

The HIV/AIDS pandemic is exacerbated by conditions of violence and instability, which increase the risk of exposure to the diseases through large movements of people, widespread uncertainty over conditions, and reduced access to medical care . . . If unchecked, the HIV/AIDS pandemic may pose a risk to stability and security.

Source: UN Security Council Resolution 1308 (17 July 2000) as quoted in UNAIDS. *HIV/AIDS and Security*. UNAIDS Fact Sheet. August 2003.

TABLE 3-2 HIV/AIDS Cases in the Russian Military, 1991–2004

Year	Cumulative Total
1991	4
1992	6
1993	8
1994	15
1995	17
1996	46
1997	118
1998	164
1999	281
2000	391
2001	1,132
2002	1,686
2003	2,067
2004	2,188

Source: Data from Murray Feshbach, "HIV/AIDS in the Russian Military–Update," Prepared for UNAIDS Meeting, Copenhagen, Denmark, February (2005).

BOX 3-5 Disease, Security, Foreign Policy, and Diplomacy

In 1978, Peter Bourne, then the Special Assistant to President Carter for Health Issues, completed a study on international health policy and called for a diplomatic strategy to both improve global health and utilize health efforts to affect foreign policy. In recent years, this concept of health and its relationship to foreign policy and opportunities for diplomacy has been reinvigorated. There is still much debate over exactly how and when global health efforts affect foreign policy and whether the health concern needs to also be a security concern in order to raise its importance in policy circles. But there is a growing recognition of the opportunities presented by health diplomacy and the importance of significantly contributing to efforts to detect, control, and treat diseases around the world.

Sources: Bourne PG. A partnership for international health care. *Public Health Reports.* March–April 1978;93(2):114–123; Feldbaum H, Michaud J. Health diplomacy and the enduring relevance of foreign policy interests. *PLoS Medicine.* April 2010;7(4); and Fidler DP. Eastphalia emerging?: Asia, international law, and global governance. *Indiana Journal of Global Legal Studies.* Winter 2010;17(1):1–12.

The United States has also engaged in relationship building and health diplomacy to further both health and foreign relations, as discussed in **Box 3-5**.

Domestic efforts have focused on improving surveillance, research, countermeasures and diagnostics, surge capacity for catastrophic events, and community resilience. These topics will all be addressed throughout the course of this book.

KEY WORDS

Health security
SARS
HIV/AIDS
Monkeypox
Health diplomacy

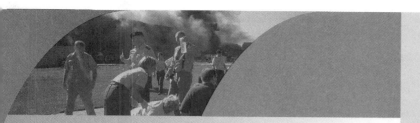

Discussion Questions

1. What is health security?

2. Why and when is a natural infectious disease a security threat? To whom?

3. Can chronic disease be a security threat? Explain the relationship.

4. How does urbanization in one part of the world become a security interest in others?

5. Is it necessary to securitize a health issue to gain political support to direct resources to the global community?

6. Can you think of an example of "health diplomacy"?

7. Should health be used as a diplomatic tool?

8. Are there any detriments to making disease a security issue?

REFERENCES

1. Weber AC. Assistant to the Secretary of Defense for Nuclear and Chemical and Biological Defense Programs. *Second Annual Richard and Janet Southby Distinguished Lectureship in Comparative Health Policy.* The George Washington University School of Public Health and Health Services; Washington, DC; April 6, 2010.

2. Frenk J, Dean's Message: H1N1 and Comprehensive Health Security—Health Reform in an Era of Pandemics. *Harvard School of Public Health.* Winter 2010. Available at: http://www.hsph.harvard.edu/news/hphr/winter-2010/winter10frenk.html. Accessed July 25, 2010.

3. U.S. Department of Health and Human Services. *National Health Security Strategy of The United States of America.* December 2009. Available at: http://www.phe.gov/Preparedness/planning/authority/nhss/strategy/Documents/nhss-final.pdf. Accessed July 25, 2010.

4. Fidler DP. From International sanitary conventions to global health security: The new international health regulations. *Chinese Journal of International Law.* 2005;4(2):325–392.

5. World Health Organization. *The World Health Report 2007: A Safer Future—Global Public Health Security in the 21st Century.* 2007.

6. Barry JM. *The Great Influenza: The Epic Story of the Deadliest Plague in History*: Penguin Books; 2005.

7. Clinton WJ. Presidential Decision Directive NSTC-7. *Federation of American Scientists.* 1996. Available at: http://www.fas.org/irp/offdocs/pdd/pdd-nstc-7.pdf. Accessed July 25, 2010.

8. The White House, Office of the Vice President. Vice President Announces Policy on Infectious Diseases. *Federation of American Scientists.* June 12, 1996. Available at: http://www.fas.org/irp/offdocs/pdd_ntsc7.htm. Accessed July 25, 2010.

9. National Intelligence Council. The Global infectious disease threat and its implications for the United States. *National Intelligence Estimate.* January 2000. Available at: http://www.dni.gov/nic/PDF_GIF_otherprod/infectiousdisease/infectiousdiseases.pdf. Accessed July 25, 2010.

10. United Nations Security Council. Security Council Resolution 1308: On the Responsibility of the Security Council in the Maintenance of International Peace and Security: HIV/AIDS and International Peacekeeping Operations. *Security Council Resolutions—2000.* July 17, 2000. Available at: http://daccess-dds-ny.un.org/doc/UNDOC/GEN/N00/536/02/PDF/N0053602.pdf?OpenElement. Accessed July 25, 2010.

11. Gellman B. AIDS is declared threat to security. *The Washington Post.* April 2000:A01; Available at: http://www.washingtonpost.com/ac2/wp-dyn?pagename=article&node=&contentId=A40503-2000Apr29. Accessed July 25, 2010.

12. The White House. *The National Security Strategy of the United States of America.* September 2002. Available at: http://georgewbush-whitehouse.archives.gov/nsc/nss/2002/. Accessed July 25, 2010.

13. The White House. *The National Security Strategy of the United States of America.* March 2006. Available at: http://georgewbush-whitehouse.archives.gov/nsc/nss/2006/. Accessed July 25, 2010.

14. The White House. *National Security Strategy.* May 2010. Available at: http://www.whitehouse.gov/sites/default/files/rss_viewer/national_security_strategy.pdf. Accessed July 25, 2010.

15. Medical Follow-Up Agency (MFUA); Institute of Medicine (IOM). Introduction and history—Naturally occurring infectious diseases in the U.S. military. In: Lemon SM, Thaul S, Fisseha S, O'Maon HC, eds. *Protecting Our Forces: Improving Vaccine Acquisition and Availability in the U.S. Military.* Washington, DC: The National Academies Press; 2002. Available at: http://www.nap.edu/openbook.php?record_id=10483&page=9.

16. Murry CK, Hinkle MK, Yun HC. History of infections associated with combat-related injuries. *The Journal of Trauma—Injury, Infection, & Critical Care.* March 2008;64(3):S221–S231. Available at: http://afids.org/Prevention%20and%20Management%20of%20CRI%20(4)%20-%20History.pdf.

17. Writer JV, DeFraites RF, Keep LW. Non-battle injury casualties during the Persian Gulf War and other deployments. *American Journal of Preventive Medicine.* April 2000;18(3, Supplement 1):64–70.

18. *Global Emerging Infections Surveillance and Response Systems (GEIS) Operations.* Armed Forces Health Surveillance Center. Available at: http://www.afhsc.mil/geis. Accessed July 25, 2010.

19. Walter Reed Army Institute of Research. *U.S. Army Medical Research and Materiel Command.* Available at: http://wrair-www.army.mil/. Accessed July 25, 2010.

20. U.S. Department of State. *Infectious and Chronic Disease.* Available at: http://www.state.gov/g/oes/intlhealthbiodefense/id/index.htm. Accessed August 1, 2010.

21. National Intelligence Council. *Strategic Implications of Global Health.* December 2008. Available at: http://www.dni.gov/nic/PDF_GIF_otherprod/ICA_Global_Health_2008.pdf. Accessed July 25, 2010.

22. The White House, Office of the Press Secretary. Statement by the President on Global Health Initiative. May 5, 2009. Available at: http://www.whitehouse.gov/the_press_office/Statement-by-the-President-on-Global-Health-Initiative/. Accessed August 1, 2010.

23. Centers for Disease Control and Prevention. Update: Multistate outbreak of monkeypox—Illinois, Indiana, Kansas, Missouri, Ohio, and Wisconsin, 2003. *Morbidity and Mortality Weekly Report.* July 2003;52(27):642–646.

24. Reynolds G. Why were doctors afraid to treat Rebecca McLester? [so they called-in doctors Michael and Stephanie Anderson who both stepped-up.]. *Children's Pediatric Center—East Main.* April 18, 2004. Available at: http://www.childrenspediatrics.com/monkey_pox.htm. Accessed August 1, 2010.

25. Institute of Medicine. *Learning from SARS: Preparing for the Next Disease Outbreak.* Washington, DC: The National Academies Press; 2004. Available at http://www.nap.edu/catalog.php?record_id=10915.

26. U.S. Department of Health and Human Services, Centers for Disease Control and Prevention. Update: Outbreak of severe acute respiratory syndrome—worldwide, 2003. *Morbidity and Mortality Weekly Report.* March 2003;52(12):241–248.

27. Olsen SJ, Chang HL, Cheung TYY, et al. Transmission of the severe acute respiratory syndrome on aircraft. *The New England Journal of Medicine.* December 2003;349(25):2416–2422.

28. National Intelligence Council. *SARS: Down But Still a Threat.* August 2003. Available at: http://www.dni.gov/nic/PDF_GIF_otherprod/sarsthreat/56797book.pdf. Accessed August 1, 2010.

29. UNAIDS. *2008 Report on the Global AIDS Epidemic.* UNAIDS; August 2008.

30. Waal A. HIV/AIDS and the challenges of security and conflict. *The Lancet.* January 2010;375(9708):22–23.

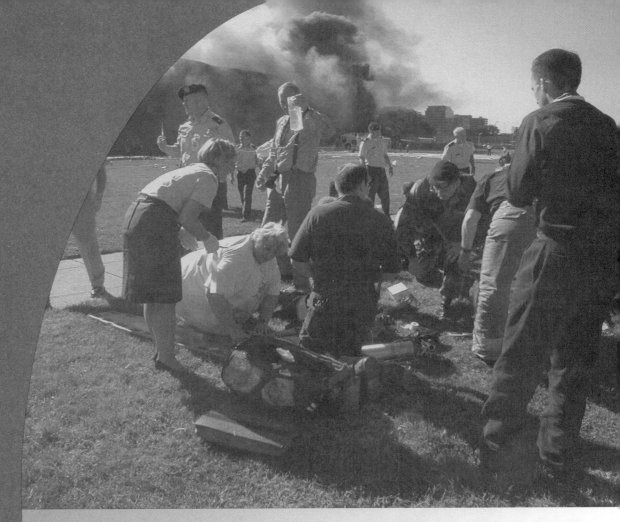

PART III

Infrastructure

CHAPTER 4

September 11, 2001 and Its Aftermath

LEARNING OBJECTIVES

By the end of this chapter, the reader will be able to:

- Understand the origins of the preparedness regime.
- Review the immediate response to the 9/11 disaster.
- Characterize the offices, organizations, and policies that emerged in the aftermath of 9/11.
- Become familiar with the intelligence community.

INTRODUCTION

The public health community does not operate in a vacuum, and public health preparedness, in particular, functions within a large, relatively new, and often shifting infrastructure of organizations and policies. In this chapter, we will review the federal government's role in preparedness and response, how it has developed over time, and the shifts that occurred after the September 11, 2001, terrorist disaster. We also look at the offices, organizations, and policies that have emerged in the past decade that relate directly to public health preparedness. Finally, this chapter introduces readers to the intelligence community (IC). In the past, the public health community had minimal interaction with the IC. While most local and state public health professionals still do not interface with this community, many federal public health professionals working on preparedness have begun to coordinate with their IC colleagues. This community, though, is foreign to most public health professionals; therefore, this chapter will provide an overview of the organizations within the community and some of the basic concepts associated with intelligence.

CONSTITUTIONAL FRAMEWORK AND HISTORY OF FEDERAL ASSISTANCE FOR PREPAREDNESS AND DISASTER RESPONSE

Under the U.S. Constitution, powers are delegated to both the federal and state governments. Under this arrangement, state and local governments are responsible for public health and safety from domestic threats (including natural threats).[1(10th amend.)] The federal government is responsible for protection from external threats or protection from internal rebellion.[1(Art. I §§ 8–10, Art. II § 2, Art. IV § 4)]* Following this delineation, the federal government had only a supportive role in disaster response, with the state and local governments responsible for preparedness and response. According to Foster, there were both practical and philosophical reasons for the limited federal role. The practical reasons prior to the Civil War included a very small federal government, with almost all of its workforce located in Washington, D.C., and limited infrastructure to support the logistics involved in sending relief and supplies to an affected region.[2,3(p 4)] The philosophical rationale for a limited federal role in disaster response was based on the prevailing concept of self-help and, if need be, assistance from private organizations, as opposed to government aid.

In 1803, Congress passed the first law related to domestic disaster assistance. (See **Box 4-1**.) This act came after

---

* Note that the U.S. Constitution contains no provision ensuring federal assistance during a disaster. Although the federal government may assist, the Tenth Amendment does reserve to the states those powers not specifically enumerated.

BOX 4-1 Text of the 1803 Federal Domestic Disaster Aid Bill, from January 14, 1803

A Bill for the Relief of Sufferers by Fire, in the town of Portsmouth

Be it enacted, by the Senate and House of Representatives of the United States of America, in Congress assembled, That the Secretary of the Treasury be, and he hereby is authorized and directed to cause to be suspended for months, the collection of bonds due to the United States by merchants of Portsmouth, in New Hampshire, who have suffered by the late conflagration of that town.

Source: 1803 Federal Domestic Disaster Aid Bill, from January 14, 1803.

Portsmouth, New Hampshire, experienced massive fires in late December 1802. The assistance was in the form of long-term financial aid as opposed to immediate assistance.[2] Congress acted similarly in response to subsequent disasters, but there was no attempt to create a comprehensive policy for federal disaster assistance or preparedness. Between 1803 and 1950, Congress passed legislation to provide relief in 128 separate natural disaster instances. Over time, the assistance shifted from financial aid (relief from bond payments) to in-kind assistance.[4]

After the Civil War, there was a shift in how the federal government perceived its responsibilities toward disaster relief, as well as a greater willingness (and need) on the part of individuals to ask for assistance. In March 1865, Congress created the Freedmen's Bureau, located administratively within the War Department. The purpose of the organization was to aid former slaves, and it took on multiple projects, including land reform, labor practices, and the development of social institutions. It also provided relief in the form of shelter and supplies to refugees and freedmen.[5] Through the Freedmen's Bureau, the army became the federal asset tasked with providing disaster relief.

Federal disaster assistance had become not only popular but also expected, and in the 1930s the Reconstruction Finance Corporation became responsible for providing loans for disaster recovery. Other federal agencies were given more authority to assist in both disaster response and preparedness. This was done on a piecemeal basis and not as part of a comprehensive approach to preparedness or response.[6] In

1953, President Harry Truman issued Executive Order 10427, which emphasized that federal assistance was only to supplement, not supplant, state, local, and private organizations' resources in response to disasters. President Richard Nixon restated and supported this in 1973.[7] By the late 1970s, there were more than 100 federal agencies involved in some aspect of disaster preparedness and response—yet, the policy firmly stated that the federal government was only to assist state and local entities, who were in charge. The National Governor's Association asked President Jimmy Carter to centralize federal government functions, and Carter responded in 1979 with Executive Order 12127, which created the Federal Emergency Management Agency (FEMA).[6,8]

In 1974, Congress passed the Disaster Relief Act,[9] which created a process for presidential disaster declarations, as a requirement to trigger financial and physical assistance from FEMA for any domestic disaster. In 1988, the Stafford Disaster Relief and Emergency Assistance Act (Stafford Act)[10] amended the Disaster Relief Act and became the principal document for federal authority and dispersal of funds for assisting state and local governments in responding to any type of disaster. This act mandates that the governor of a state make a formal request to the president to declare either a major disaster or an emergency. (See **Box 4-2**.) Once the declaration is made, FEMA is then responsible for coordinating relief efforts across 28 federal agencies and nongovernmental organizations, including the American Red Cross. The Stafford Act has been amended several times, including passage of the Disaster Mitigation Act in 2000[11] and the Pets Evacuation and Transportation Standards Act in 2006.[12] **Figure 4-1** depicts when and how federal resources are deployed during a disaster.

The 1995 Presidential Decision Directive 39 (PDD-39), "United States Policy on Counterterrorism," was the last major policy guideline that addressed disaster preparedness and response. This directive reaffirmed that FEMA would be in charge of consequence management during an emergency—including any terrorist event—while the FBI would handle crisis management for threats or acts of terrorism within the United States. (See **Figure 4-2**.) All other federal agencies would provide support where appropriate under coordination by the National Security Council.

IMMEDIATE RESPONSE TO 9/11

Prior to 2001, as we have discussed, plans and policies were in place for federal response efforts, primarily designed for natural disasters. The federal government had always taken a position of assisting state and local agencies, not running a disaster response. On September 11, 2001, the United States experienced a major terrorist disaster, which forced a para-

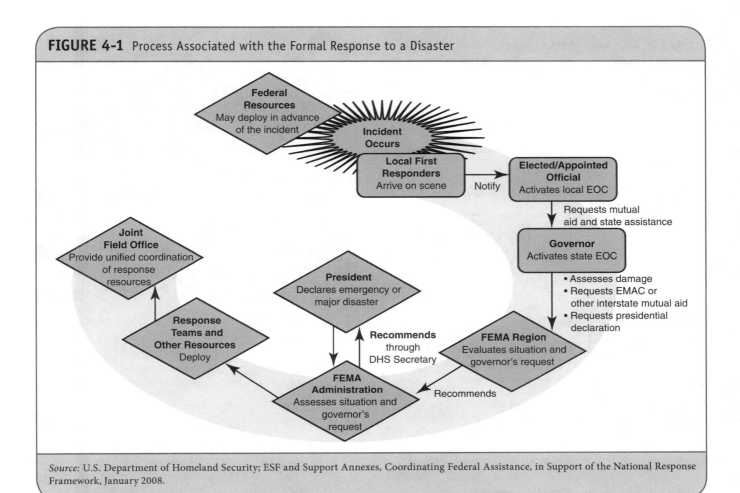

FIGURE 4-1 Process Associated with the Formal Response to a Disaster

Source: U.S. Department of Homeland Security; ESF and Support Annexes, Coordinating Federal Assistance, in Support of the National Response Framework, January 2008.

digm shift in thinking about federal responsibilities. This was a major national emergency and was not caused by a natural disaster. This was a disaster related to national security in an arena where the federal government is responsible for "providing for the common defense." Many were forced to rethink how they conceive of disasters, federal roles, national security, and a new term that entered the vocabulary—homeland security.

In November 2002, the National Commission on Terrorist Attacks Upon the United States was convened to review the events leading up to the 9/11 attacks and to make recommendations for moving forward. The Commission's final report was released in July 2004 and is known as the *9/11 Commission Report*. The Commission found "the 9/11 attacks revealed four kinds of failures: in imagination, policy, capabilities, and management," which led to the events of 9/11.[13(p 339)] On *imagination*, many in government and across the country did not give adequate consideration to the possibility of a foreign terrorist attack on U.S. soil. On *policy*, terrorism was not a major pri-

ority for either the Clinton or the (pre-9/11) George W. Bush administration. It was considered and there was expertise devoted to it but not nearly enough given the true threat. On *capabilities*, the United States operated in a Cold War mind-set, focusing on past threats instead of thinking about future conflicts. Military and intelligence organizations were not concentrating on a terrorist threat. There was very little convergence between local FBI agents and national priorities. The Federal Aviation Administration was not strong enough. On *management*, the Commission found an inability on the part of the federal government to manage new problems. Not enough information was shared among agencies, duties were not clearly assigned, and there was limited management of how top leaders set priorities and allocated resources, particularly within the intelligence community.

One major finding of the *9/11 Commission Report* was that the U.S. federal government did not have a fully integrated, communicative, functional homeland security infrastructure, including emergency preparedness, which includes

FIGURE 4-2 PDD 39 from 1995: Relationship Among Federal Agencies for Cases and Consequence Management in Response to Terrorist Acts

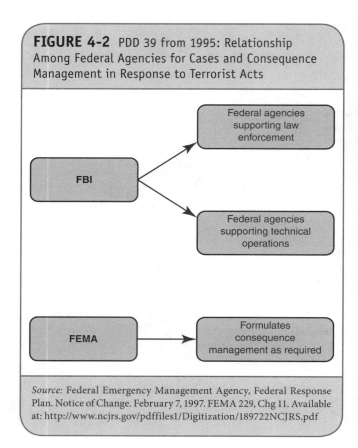

Source: Federal Emergency Management Agency, Federal Response Plan. Notice of Change. February 7, 1997. FEMA 229, Chg 11. Available at: http://www.ncjrs.gov/pdffiles1/Digitization/189722NCJRS.pdf

everything from first responders to public health infrastructure. **Box 4-3** details some of the challenges and failures of the U.S. government leading up to September 11, 2001.

POST-9/11

Almost immediately after 9/11 and the release of the *9/11 Commission Report* the United States began to make a series of changes, resulting in the most massive reorganization of the federal government since World War II. The following are some of the initial changes:

- *Executive Order 13228, October 8, 2001:* Established the Office of Homeland Security and the Homeland Security Council. Executive Order 13228 was the first effort by President George W. Bush following the 9/11 attacks. It established an Office of Homeland Security within the White House and directed that the assistant to the president for Homeland Security should be the individual primarily responsible for coordinating the domestic response efforts of all departments and agencies in the event of an imminent terrorist threat and immediately following an attack. Tom Ridge, the former governor of Pennsylvania, was appointed to fill this position.

BOX 4-2 Robert T. Stafford Disaster Relief and Emergency Assistance Act, Public Law 93-288, as amended, 42 U.S.C. 5121–5207, and Related Authorities Title I—Findings, Declarations, and Definitions Sec. 101. Congressional Findings and Declarations (42 U.S.C. 5121)

It is the intent of the Congress, by this Act, to provide an orderly and continuing means of assistance by the Federal Government to State and local governments in carrying out their responsibilities to alleviate the suffering and damage which result from such disasters by—

(1) revising and broadening the scope of existing disaster relief programs;

(2) encouraging the development of comprehensive disaster preparedness and assistance plans, programs, capabilities, and organizations by the States and by local governments;

(3) achieving greater coordination and responsiveness of disaster preparedness and relief programs;

(4) encouraging individuals, States, and local governments to protect themselves by obtaining insurance coverage to supplement or replace governmental assistance;

(5) encouraging hazard mitigation measures to reduce losses from disasters, including development of land use and construction regulations; and

(6) providing Federal assistance programs for both public and private losses sustained in disasters

Source: FEMA 592, June 2007 (42 U.S.C. 5121).

- *National Security Presidential Directive 8 (NSPD 8), 2001:* With the establishment of the office and council of Homeland Security came the creation of the position of the national director and deputy national security

BOX 4-3 *9/11 Commission Report* Findings: The United States Government Challenges and Failures Leading up to September 11, 2001

Unsuccessful Diplomacy

- As early as February 1997, the U.S. government attempted to use diplomatic pressure to convince different states to cease support to al Qaeda and Osama Bin Laden, including the Taliban regime in Afghanistan, Pakistan, and the United Arab Emirates. These attempts included incentives, sanctions, and even warnings of retribution, but the United States could not find the right balance between these approaches, and diplomatic attempts were largely fruitless.

Lack of Military Options

- In the summer of 1998, policy makers requested the military, prepare options for conducting an attack on Bin Laden and al Qaeda. A great emphasis was placed on the need for actionable intelligence before launching any strike. The lack of such intelligence tied the hands of the military and frustrated policy makers, as they could not risk the possibility of inflicting serious collateral damage and could not afford to have any attack fail because either scenario would make Bin Laden appear strong and the United States weak.

Problems within the Intelligence Community

- Due to competing priorities, budget constraints, an inefficient structure, and typical bureaucratic rivalries, the intelligence community's effort to combat transnational terrorism was inadequate. Not only was there a lack of any comprehensive review of what the Central Intelligence Agency (CIA) knew or did not know on the matter, it was also limited to using proxies in its efforts to disrupt terrorist activities by capturing Bin Laden or his lieutenants, which produced a frustrating lack of results.

Problems within the FBI

- Following the first terrorist attack on the World Trade Center in 1993, the FBI became increasingly involved in the counterterrorism effort. However, its resources were primarily devoted to investigating and prosecuting terrorists after attacks, not preventing them from happening in the first place. Efforts to change this policy were fairly unsuccessful, mostly due to the FBI's bureaucratically limited capacity or its reluctance to share information.

Permeable Borders and Immigration Controls

- Intelligence and law enforcement officials were both presented with opportunities to prevent al Qaeda's attacks by exploiting their travel vulnerabilities since the 9/11 participants included known al Qaeda operatives who both behaved suspiciously and presented suspicious paperwork. Prior to the 9/11 attacks, however, protecting national borders was not a priority, and the Immigration and Naturalization Service was not considered a partner in the counterterrorism effort.

Permeable Aviation Security

- The hijackers in the 9/11 attack only needed to get past the security checkpoint process to carry out their attacks, an obstacle easily overcome by simply studying publicly available materials on the subject. After some of the hijackers were selected for extra screening, the only action taken was a more highly scrutinized examination of their checked baggage.

Financing

- The 9/11 attacks cost between $400,000 and $500,000 to execute, making them extremely economical attacks. The operatives' transactions were not suspicious and were effectively invisible amid the billions of daily purchases in the United States.

An Improvised Homeland Defense

- Both the Federal Aviation Administration (FAA) and North American Aerospace Defense Command (NORAD) were unprepared for the type of attack launched against the United States on 9/11. Both implemented the best course of action possible given the information at hand, but communication at more senior levels was poor. The military and the FAA had little to no communication with each other, and senior officials of the president's staff, such as the secretary of defense, were not brought into the chain of command until the key events of the morning had already occurred.

Source: National Commission on Terrorist Attacks Upon the United States; *The 9/11 Commission Report.*

advisor for combating terrorism, tasked with operational coordination of combating transnational terrorist activities.

- *Homeland Security Act of 2002, passed in 2003:* This act created the Department of Homeland Security, reorganizing multiple existing agencies under a single department, as well as creating new responsibilities for security and preparedness.
- A series of Homeland Security Presidential Directives (HSPDs), aimed at national preparedness, and response policies and guidance documents were issued. (Chapter 5 will provide more information on these HSPDs, and **Box 4-4** helps define the different types of presidential directives, including HSPDs.)

In July 2002, the George W. Bush administration released the National Strategy for Homeland Security, which identified six critical mission areas: intelligence and warning, border and transportation security, domestic counterterrorism, protecting critical infrastructure and key assets, defending against catastrophic events, and emergency preparedness and response. While the public health community is not directly referenced in this strategy (although emergency medical providers are identified as America's first line of defense in the aftermath of an attack),[14(p 41)] public health contributes to at least three of the six critical mission areas: (1) intelligence—disease surveillance and development of medical intelligence; (2) defending against catastrophic events—improving sensor and decontamination techniques, developing vaccines and medical countermeasures, harnessing scientific knowledge and tools to counter terrorism, and controlling access to dangerous agents; and (3) emergency preparedness and response—preparing the healthcare community for catastrophic terrorism, augmenting medical countermeasure supplies, preparing for decontamination needs, building volunteer systems, enhancing victim support systems, preparing hospitals for surge capacity, training and deploying disaster medical assistance teams, and preparing first responders to work safely in areas where dangerous weapons have been used.

OFFICES AND ORGANIZATIONS: THE FEDERAL PREPAREDNESS INFRASTRUCTURE

In addition to the creation of the Department of Homeland Security in the wake of 9/11, many existing organizations established new offices, expanded existing ones, and redirected resources toward preparedness and homeland security. Here are the offices and organizations most directly linked to public health preparedness.

BOX 4-4 Overview of Presidential Directives

The president uses several instruments to establish, continue, or cease federal policies. Here are some of the most common directives, including those referenced in this textbook.

Executive Order [EO]: A presidential directive with the authority of a law, an executive order directs and governs action by executive officials and agencies.

Homeland Security Presidential Directives [HSPDs]: Following 9/11, the Bush administration created the Homeland Security Council, which then released a series of directives to record and communicate presidential decisions and policies related to homeland security in the United States.

National Security Council Directives: Different administrations have had their own names for national security directives used for decision and review of national security policies and strategies. These are a type of executive order but done with the advice and consent of the National Security Council. Like EOs, they have the effect of law. Nomenclatures used by different administrations include:

- **National Security Decision Directive (NSDD)**—Reagan.
- **National Security Directive (NSD)**—G. H. W. Bush.
- **Presidential Decision Directive (PDD)**—Clinton.
- **National Security Presidential Directive (NSPD)**—G. W. Bush.
- **Presidential Policy Directive (PPD)**—Obama.

Source: Relyea H. *Presidential Directives: Background and Overview.* CRS Report for Congress. November 26, 2008.

Department of Health and Human Services (DHHS)

Office of the Assistant Secretary for Preparedness and Response (ASPR)

The Pandemic and All-Hazards Preparedness Act of 2006 created the Office of the Assistant Secretary, and replaced the office previously known as the Office of Public Health Emergency Preparedness. ASPR is composed of multiple components, including the Biomedical Advanced Research and Development Authority (BARDA), the Office of Preparedness and Emergency Operations, and Policy and Planning. ASPR is responsible for "preventing, preparing for, and responding to adverse health effects of public health emergencies and disasters."[15] In addition to policy development, the office supports state and local capacity during emergencies by providing federal support. This includes deployment of clinicians through the National Disaster Medical System.

Centers for Disease Control and Prevention (CDC)

The Centers for Disease Control and Prevention has consolidated its preparedness activities under the Office of Public Health Preparedness and Response. This office coordinates and responds to public health threats through a multitude of programs, including an emergency operations division that constantly maintains situational awareness of potential threats; a division dedicated to supporting preparedness at the state, local, tribal, and territorial levels through cooperative agreements, providing approximately $7 billion to date toward preparedness efforts for all hazard threats; a division that hosts and manages the strategic national stockpile of medical countermeasures and supplies necessary to address a large-scale public health emergency; and a division devoted to regulating the select agent program.

National Institutes of Health (NIH)

The National Institutes of Health is engaged in public health preparedness through a variety of offices. The two primary locations are the Office of Science Policy, which houses the National Science Advisory Board for Biosecurity (NSABB). Additionally, the National Institute of Allergy and Infectious Diseases (NIAID) hosts a robust research agenda, both intramural and in support of extramural programs, that supports the research and development of medical countermeasures against radiological, nuclear, and chemical threats and supports biodefense activities.[16]

The Food and Drug Administration (FDA)

The Food and Drug Administration has multiple offices that address emergency preparedness and response. These offices focus on regulatory oversight, monitoring infrastructure, and facilitating the delivery of appropriate countermeasures. Specifically, the Office of Crisis Management coordinates emergency and crisis response, as related to FDA-regulated products. The Center for Biologics and Evaluation Research oversees safety and effectiveness of biologic products, includ-

ing CBRN medical countermeasures. The Office of Counterterrorism and Emerging Threats works on policies, strategies, and interagency communication around counterterrorism. It also coordinates activities around emergency use authorization for medical countermeasures.[17]

Department of Homeland Security (DHS)

The main office within DHS that addresses public health preparedness is the Office of Health Affairs. This office has four main branches. The Weapons of Mass Destruction and Biodefense Office oversees biodefense activities, including Project Bioshield and bio-aerosol environmental monitoring systems. The Medical Readiness Office works with the first responder community, provides health and medical security issues during emergencies, and oversees health components of contingency planning for CBRN. The Component Services Office focuses on occupational health and safety, workforce health protection, and medical services for DHS. Lastly, the International Affairs and Global Health Security office provides expertise on health security and emergency planning and coordinates information sharing with global and private-sector partners.[18]

The Science and Technology Directorate houses the Chemical and Biological Division, which works on threat awareness, surveillance and detection, and countermeasures. This directorate also is home to the Office of National Laboratories, which includes a series of major research labs that support biodefense; microbial forensics; and basic understandings of chemical, biological, and agricultural threats.

FEMA is also within DHS. We will discuss the role of FEMA in detail in subsequent chapters, particularly its coordination role for responding to emergencies.

Department of Agriculture (USDA)

The Animal and Plant Health Inspection Service (APHIS) at USDA has a broad mission to protect and promote U.S. agricultural health. APHIS also works with DHS and FEMA to provide assistance and coordination during emergencies. This assistance ranges from disease containment in poultry, such as in cases of avian influenza, to protecting health of livestock and crops from foreign disease.[19]

Department of Justice, Federal Bureau of Investigation (FBI)

The Federal Bureau of Investigation created a new WMD Directorate in 2006. This directorate works in several areas, including countermeasures and preparedness, investigations and operations, and intelligence analysis. The investigative component directs the WMD threat credibility assessments and manages all WMD criminal investigations. On preparedness, the FBI works with field components, as well as with other agencies. In particular, the FBI works closely with CDC on "Crim-Epi," the cooperation between law enforcement and epidemiologists in the investigation of potential WMD events in a way that enables the FBI to collect information that will lead to a prosecution but that also enables epidemiologists to investigate, treat, and minimize morbidity and mortality.[20]

Department of Defense

The Department of Defense (DoD) has a massive infrastructure designed to address threats of any nature, including public health emergencies. The military is trained in emergency response and preparedness as critical components of an effective military. While many DoD programs focus on protecting the war fighter, several also have implications for the broader civilian population, including the programs that fall under stability operations. There is an active chemical and biological defense program that involves research, development, and testing defense systems and equipment, including medical countermeasures. The Cooperative Threat Reduction Programs work to reduce the threat of WMDs, while building global capacity for detection and response to biological threats. There is a large-scale laboratory network both in the United States and abroad engaged in basic scientific research for infectious diseases, as well as epidemiologic response to public health emergencies. For emergency response within the United States, U.S. Northern Command (USNORTHCOM) has the lead within DoD and is charged with coordinating DoD support to civilian authorities. There are several consequence management response teams, including those specifically trained to respond to WMD events.[21]

While the Department of Defense has many assets that can contribute to emergency preparedness and response to public health events, it must act within the limits of the Posse Comitatus Act (see **Box 4-5**). Posse Comitatus is an 1878 federal law intended to limit the ability of the federal government to use the military for civilian law enforcement.[22] The act applies to the army, navy, marines, air force, and state National Guard forces but only when they are called in for federal duty. It does not apply to the Coast Guard. In 2006, in the wake of Hurricane Katrina and under pressure from President Bush, Congress passed a law that allows the use of the armed forces in major public emergencies to restore public order and enforce laws.[23](Sec. 1076) These changes to Posse Comitatus, however, were repealed by the National Defense Authorization Act for fiscal year 2008, and the original language stands.

BOX 4-5 Posse Comitatus Act

18 U.S.C. § 1385. *Use of Army and Air Force as posse comitatus*

Whoever, except in cases and under circumstances expressly authorized by the Constitution or Act of Congress, willfully uses any part of the Army or the Air Force as a posse comitatus or otherwise to execute the laws shall be fined under this title or imprisoned not more than two years, or both.

Source: 18 U.S.C. § 1385.

INTRODUCTION TO THE INTELLIGENCE COMMUNITY

A primary recommendation of the *9/11 Commission Report* was the need to unify intelligence and knowledge and create a director of national intelligence to oversee all of the intelligence community. This recommendation led to just that—a director of national intelligence (DNI), along with the creation of multiple intelligence entities within other agencies, including a Department of Defense Counterintelligence Field Activity, the Joint Intelligence Task Force for Combating Terrorism, the Office of Intelligence Analysis at the Department of the Treasury, and the National Security Services at the FBI.

The intelligence community supports policy makers, but it does not make policy or advocate for one policy choice over another. The community is an executive function of the federal government composed of multiple agencies and offices from across the executive branch. The legislative branch provides oversight committees.

At the top of the intelligence community is the National Security Council (NSC). The NSC is chaired by the president, with regular participants, including the vice president; the secretaries of state, treasury, and defense; the assistant to the president for national security affairs; the chair of the Joint Chiefs of Staff; and the director of national intelligence.

The National Security Council oversees the director of national intelligence, and the DNI oversees the rest of the intelligence community, including the Central Intelligence Agency. Under the DNI, there are 10 mission support activities:

- National Counterterrorism Center (NCTC).
- National Counterintelligence Executive (NCIX).
- National Counterproliferation Center (NCPC).
- Special Security Center (SCC).

- National Intelligence University (NIU).
- Intelligence Advanced Research Projects Activity (IARPA).
- Center for Security Evaluation (CSE).
- National Intelligence Council (NIC).
- National Intelligence Coordination Center (NIC-C).
- Mission Support Center.

Under the DNI there are 16 members that make up the rest of the intelligence community. The only independent agency in this community is the Central Intelligence Agency.

BOX 4-6 Intelligence Community Members

- **Independent agency**
  - Central Intelligence Agency (CIA)
- **Department of Defense (DoD)**
  - **Agencies/offices**
    - Defense Intelligence Agency (DIA)
    - National Geospatial-Intelligence Agency (NGA)
    - National Reconnaissance Office (NRO)
    - National Security Agency (NSA)
  - **Service components**
    - Air Force Intelligence, Surveillance and Reconnaissance Agency
    - Army Military Intelligence
    - Marine Corps Intelligence Activity
    - Office of Naval Intelligence
- **Department of Energy**
  - Office of Intelligence and Counterintelligence
- **Department of Homeland Security**
  - Office of Intelligence and Analysis (IA)
  - Coast Guard Intelligence and Criminal Investigations Program
- **Department of Justice**
  - Drug Enforcement Administration, Office of National Security Intelligence (DEA)
  - Federal Bureau of Investigation, Directorate of Intelligence
- **Department of State**
  - Bureau of Intelligence and Research (INR)
- **Department of the Treasury**
  - Office of Intelligence and Analysis

The other 15 elements, shown in **Box 4-6**, are offices, bureaus, or agencies situated within executive branch departments.

Each member of the intelligence community tailors its work to the specific needs of its customers, specifically the priorities of the home agency. The entire IC, however, uses the same set of terminology. There are six major types of intelligence utilized by the IC, with some members of the community focusing more on some types than others:

1. *Human Intelligence (HUMINT)*—HUMINT uses people to gain information. It is the oldest form of information collection.
2. *Imagery Intelligence (IMINT)*—IMINT comes from photography, sensors, electro-optics, and radar. This type of intelligence can come from land, sea, air, or space platforms.
3. *Signals Intelligence (SIGINT)*—SIGINT includes foreign communications intercepts (COMINT), technical or geolocation intelligence (ELINT), and electromagnetic radiation and electrically transmitted data intercepts (FISINT).
4. *Measurement and Signature Intelligence (MASINT)*—MASINT is the quantitative and qualitative analysis of data coming from technical sensors.
5. *Open Source Intelligence (OSINT)*—OSINT is the exploitation of news media and public sources for uses by the intelligence community.
6. *Technical Intelligence (TECHINT)*—TECHINT is the exploitation of foreign material.

Each member of the intelligence community produces products (papers, briefings, and the like) for its respective agency, and that information may be shared and coordinated with the DNI and even reported up to the president, depending on the need for the intelligence information to inform policy development. The community also produces national intelligence estimates under the purview of the National Intelligence Council within the DNI. These are the intelligence community's most authoritative written judgments on specific national security issues, with input from the entire community.

KEY WORDS

Stafford Act
Disaster assistance
9/11 Commission Report
Presidential directives
Intelligence community

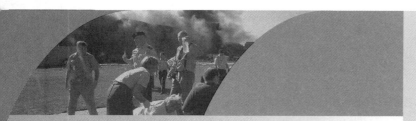

Discussion Questions

1. Describe the events that led to the redesign of the national preparedness infrastructure.

2. Do you believe there should be more or less federal involvement in state and local disaster response?

3. Given the findings from the *9/11 Commission Report*, which do you think are most important for future planning and policy development? Which most directly affect the public health community?

4. Do you think the intelligence community works well together? Does it work well with outside entities? How do you think the public health community should engage the intelligence community and, if so, how? Is there a downside for the public health community to working closely with the intelligence community?

5. Try to create an organizational chart linking all of the federal agencies associated with preparedness activities.

REFERENCES

1. Constitution of the United States of America.

2. Suburban Emergency Management Project. *History of Federal Domestic Disaster Aid Before the Civil War.* July 24, 2006. Available at: http://www.semp.us/publications/biot_reader.php?BiotID=379. Accessed August 23, 2010.

3. Foster GM. *The Demands of Humanity: Army Medical Disaster Relief.* U.S. Army Medical Department, Office of Medical History. 1983. Available at: http://history.amedd.army.mil/booksdocs/misc/disaster/default.html. Accessed August 23, 2010.

4. Hoover M. Rowboat federalism: The politics of U.S. disaster relief. *MRZine.* November 28, 2005. Available at: http://mrzine.monthlyreview.org/2005/hoover281105.html. Accessed August 23, 2010.

5. Dauber ML. The sympathetic state. *Law and History Review.* 2005;23(2):387–442.

6. U.S. Department of Homeland Security. *FEMA History.* August 11, 2010. Available at: http://www.fema.gov/about/history.shtm. Accessed August 23, 2010.

7. The White House. *The Federal Response to Hurricane Katrina Lessons Learned.* February 2006. Available at: http://library.stmarytx.edu/acadlib/edocs/katrinawh.pdf. Accessed September 10, 2010.

8. Federation of American Scientists. Executive Order 12127—Federal Emergency Management Agency. March 31, 1979. Available at: http://www.fas.org/irp/offdocs/eo/eo-12127.htm. Accessed August 23, 2010.

9. Disaster Relief Act of 1974; Public Law No. 93-288.

10. Robert T. Stafford Disaster Relief and Emergency Assistance Act (Stafford Act); Public Law No. 100-707.

11. Disaster Mitigation Act of 2000; Public Law No. 106-390.

12. Pets Evacuation and Transportation Standards Act; Public Law No. 109-308.

13. National Commission on Terrorist Attacks Upon the United States. *The 9/11 Commission Report.* Available at: http://www.9-11commission.gov/report/911Report.pdf. Accessed August 23, 2010.

14. Office of Homeland Security. *National Strategy for Homeland Security.* July 2002. Available at: http://www.dhs.gov/xlibrary/assets/nat_strat_hls.pdf.

15. U.S. Department of Health and Human Services. Office of the Assistant Secretary for Preparedness and Response (ASPR). *Public Health Emergency.* May 11, 2010. Available at: http://www.phe.gov/about/aspr/pages/default.aspx. Accessed August 23, 2010.

16. U.S. Department of Health and Human Services. *Biodefense & Related Programs.* National Institute of Allergy and Infectious Diseases. November 16, 2009. Available at: http://www.niaid.nih.gov/topics/biodefenserelated/pages/default.aspx. Accessed August 23, 2010.

17. U.S. Department of Health and Human Services. *Emergency Preparedness and Response.* U.S. Food and Drug Administration. Available at: http://www.fda.gov/EmergencyPreparedness/default.htm. Accessed August 23, 2010.

18. U.S. Department of Homeland Security. Office of Health Affairs. *U.S. Department of Homeland Security.* August 26, 2009. Available at: http://www.dhs.gov/xabout/structure/editorial_0880.shtm. Accessed August 23, 2010.

19. U.S. Department of Agriculture. *Animal and Plant Health Inspection Service.* August 23, 2010. Available at: http://www.aphis.usda.gov/. Accessed August 23, 2010.

20. U.S. Department of Justice. *Federal Bureau of Investigation.* Available at: http://www.fbi.gov/homepage.htm. Accessed August 23, 2010.

21. Sandor K. Department of Defense. In: Katz R, Zilinikas R, eds. *Encyclopedia of Bioterrorism Defense*, 2nd ed. Wiley and Sons; May 2011.

22. 18 U.S.C. 1385 (2006).

23. John Warner National Defense Authorization Act for Fiscal Year 2007; Public Law No. 109-364.

Preparedness Plans

INTRODUCTION

In the wake of 9/11, the U.S. government stepped up efforts to develop, exercise, and solidify plans to address all types of emergencies that might threaten the population. In this chapter, we follow the path for the development of these plans and delve deeper into the emergency preparedness plans that have been created and tested over the past decade. We focus primarily on federal-level plans but also look at state and local preparedness planning efforts. We will examine international preparedness activities in later chapters.

On February 28, 2003, the George W. Bush administration released Homeland Security Presidential Directive 5 (HSPD 5): Management of Domestic Incidents. The purpose of this document was to establish a single, comprehensive national incident management system, ensuring that all agencies and levels of government could work together to best respond to an emergency event. HSPD 5 called for the creation of both a National Response Plan (NRP) and a National Incident Management System (NIMS) and clarified that the initial responsibility for managing an incident lies at the state and local levels; the federal government's response is designed to

be used only when state and local resources are overwhelmed, as assessed by the state and local authorities themselves.[1]

In December 2003, Homeland Security Presidential Directive 8 (HSPD 8): National Preparedness was released, building on the concepts addressed in HSPD 5 and defining preparedness (see **Box 5-1**). HSPD 8 called for the development of a national preparedness goal that would provide effective and efficient aid from the federal government, support first responders, and establish measurable priorities and targets.[2] HSPD 8 also called for an "all-hazards approach" to preparedness planning, which refers to preparedness planning that is relevant to multiple types of disasters, including terrorist events, natural disasters, and any other large-scale emergencies.

In September 2007, the government released the National Preparedness Guidelines, defining what it means for the nation to be prepared for all hazards. The purpose of the document was to strengthen and organize national preparedness

---

BOX 5-1 Preparedness Defined

. . . the existence of plans, procedures, policies, training, and equipment necessary at the Federal, State, and local level to maximize the ability to prevent, respond to, and recover from major events. The term "readiness" is used interchangeably with preparedness.

Source: HSPD 8.

efforts, guide investment, and inform the planning process. The guidelines contained four key elements:

1. *National preparedness vision*—The national preparedness vision stated: "A nation prepared with coordinated capabilities to prevent, protect against, respond to, and recover from all hazards in a way that balances risk resources and need."[3(p 1)] The vision was designed with the understanding that preparedness only comes when multiple levels of government, private organizations, and individual citizens work together to reach a common goal.

2. *National planning scenarios*—These are 15 scenarios (listed in **Box 5-2**) that represent a broad range of natural and man-made threats designed to focus national planning, training, investments, and exercises. The scenarios engage all levels of government, as well as the private sector.

3. *Universal task list*—The universal task list (UTL) is a menu of approximately 1,600 tasks that are required to "prevent, protect against, respond to, and recover"[3(p 1)] from the events listed in the national planning scenarios.

4. *Target capabilities list*—The target capabilities list (TCL) is 37 specific capabilities that organizations and individuals at all levels of government and the private sector should collectively develop and possess to respond to emergencies.

BOX 5-2 National Planning Scenarios

- Improvised nuclear device
- Major earthquake
- Aerosol anthrax
- Major hurricane
- Pandemic influenza
- Radiological dispersal device
- Plague
- Improvised explosive device
- Blister agent
- Food contamination
- Toxic industrial chemicals
- Foreign animal disease
- Nerve agent
- Cyber attack
- Chlorine tank explosion

Source: U.S. Department of Homeland Security. *National Preparedness Guidelines.* September 2007. Available at: http://www.fema.gov/pdf/government/npg.pdf. Accessed August 23, 2010.

The rationale behind these four key elements is that they are supportive of each other. The vision sets the overall goal for preparedness. The scenarios (including chemical, biological, radiological, nuclear, explosive, food and agricultural, and cyber terrorism; natural disasters; and pandemic flu) highlight the major types of emergencies the country needs to be ready for. The UTL then delineates the tasks required to address these emergencies in a comprehensive fashion to prevent, protect, respond, and recover. Finally, the TCL guides federal, state, and local entities in developing the capabilities needed to meet the tasks that enable the government to respond to the scenarios. Of the 37 capabilities on the TCL, 8 are specific to public health and medical capabilities. These include fatality management, isolation and quarantine, mass prophylaxis, medical supplies management and distribution, medical surge capacity, public health epidemiologic investigation and laboratory testing, triage and prehospital treatment, and worker health and safety.

To test preparedness and readiness, the Department of Homeland Security (DHS), through FEMA, runs an exercise and evaluation program (known as the Homeland Security Exercise and Evaluation Program [HSEEP]). The program standardizes exercises, attempts to establish common concepts, and synchronizes all exercises across the country. Importantly, this program supports state and local jurisdictions through direct funding, training, and exercise assistance. Ideally, these exercises enable jurisdictions to assess preparedness levels and take corrective action when necessary to improve capacities to respond to emergencies, as depicted in **Figure 5-1**.

NATIONAL INCIDENT MANAGEMENT SYSTEM

One of the directives in HSPD 5 was the need for the DHS to develop and administer a National Incident Management System (NIMS). What was developed was a document that provides for standardized incident management protocols that can be used by those responding to any type of emergency at all levels of government. The document itself evolved out of a need for a common language, as well as a common framework, for managing emergencies. In the past, most jurisdictions had plans in place for responding to an emergency, but many of these plans were not consistent with the plans of other localities, which had implications for coordination and management of large-scale events that involved multiple jurisdictions and multiple levels of government.

NIMS has five major components:

FIGURE 5-1 Homeland Security Exercise and Evaluation Program (HSEEP)

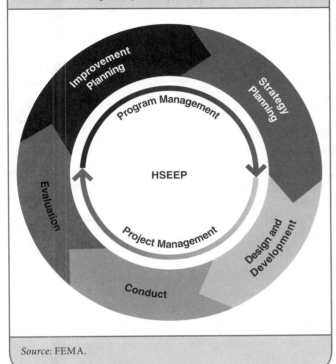

Source: FEMA.

FIGURE 5-2 National Incident Management System

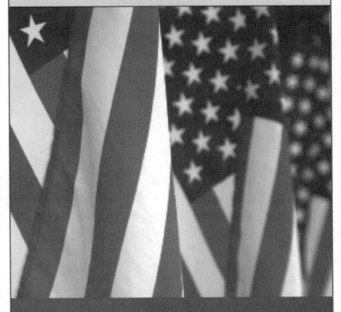

NATIONAL INCIDENT MANAGEMENT SYSTEM

December 2008

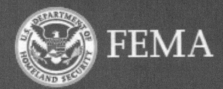 FEMA

Working together to prevent, protect against, respond to, recover from, and mitigate the effects of incidents.

Source: FEMA http://www.fema.gov/pdf/emergency/nims/NIMS_brochure.pdf

1. *Preparedness:* Establishment of guidelines and standards for planning, training, and qualifications for responders.
2. *Communications and information management:* Requirements for an interoperable communications and information process.
3. *Resource management:* Mutual-aid agreements, resource mobilization protocols, and the ability of all jurisdictional levels to access necessary resources to address an emergency.
4. *Command and management:* Standards for an incident command system, a multi-agency coordination system, and public information system.
5. *Ongoing management and maintenance:* Through the National Integration Center (NIC) and the NIMS Standards Development, maintenance of compliance, standards, and training.

Importantly, NIMS was developed as a comprehensive, systematic approach to managing an emergency that can be used at all levels of government, in every jurisdiction. It provides a common set of principles, language, and standards that can be scaled to all levels of incidents. NIMS, however, is not a specific response plan.

THE NATIONAL RESPONSE FRAMEWORK

NIMS was designed to be used in conjunction with a specific response plan, developed as the National Response Framework (NRF). (Originally, it was developed as the National Response Plan; it was revised and renamed in 2007 as the National Response Framework and revised again in 2008 (see Figure 5-3), reflecting lessons learned from past emergencies.) The NRF is a broad national plan that tries to describe the who, what, and how of preparedness and response for disasters and emergencies. It was designed to address five basic principles of response: engaged partnership, tiered response, scalable and flexible capabilities, unity of effort, and readiness to act.[4]

The NRF is organized as a core document that contains doctrines, roles and responsibilities, and planning requirements. The core document is followed by emergency support functions, support annexes, incident annexes, and partner guides. Of particular importance to the public health community is Emergency Support Function (ESF) 8, as well as the Biological Incident Annex, the Catastrophic Incident Annex, Emergency Management (ESF 5), and Oil and Hazardous Materials Response (ESF 10).

ESF 8 is devoted entirely to public health and medical services (see **Box 5-3**). This guidance document puts the Secretary of Health and Human Services in charge of public health emergencies and specifically names the assistant secretary for preparedness and response as the coordinator for ESF 8 preparedness, response, and recovery, except in emergencies that pertain to members of the armed forces. (Events involving the armed forces fall under the purview of the Department of Defense.) The purpose of ESF 8 is to provide for coordinated federal assistance for public health and medical disasters. This document addresses a number of core functional areas, including:

- Assessment of public health/medical needs.
- Health surveillance.
- Medical care personnel.
- Health/medical/veterinary equipment and supplies.
- Patient evacuation.
- Patient care.
- Safety and security of drugs, biologics, and devices.
- Food safety and security.
- Agriculture safety and security.
- Worker health safety.
- Behavioral health care.
- Public health and medical information.
- Vector control.
- Potable water and solid waste disposal.
- Fatality management (formally, victim identification/ mortuary services).[5]

In addition to ESF 8, the Biological Incident Annex outlines actions, roles, and responsibilities with regard to disease outbreaks that require federal assistance in response and containment. Department of Health and Human Services is the coordinating agency, although several other agencies take lead under particular circumstances. For example, USDA is the primary agency for outbreaks and attacks in animals that are part of commercial food production. Events that occur in wildlife fall under the purview of the Department of the Interior, and events that occur in marine animals are managed by the Department of Commerce.[6]

The goals of the Biological Incident Annex are to ensure that events are detected, the causative agent is identified, the population is protected, and the issues pertaining to re-

FIGURE 5-3 National Response Framework

National Response Framework

January 2008

Homeland Security

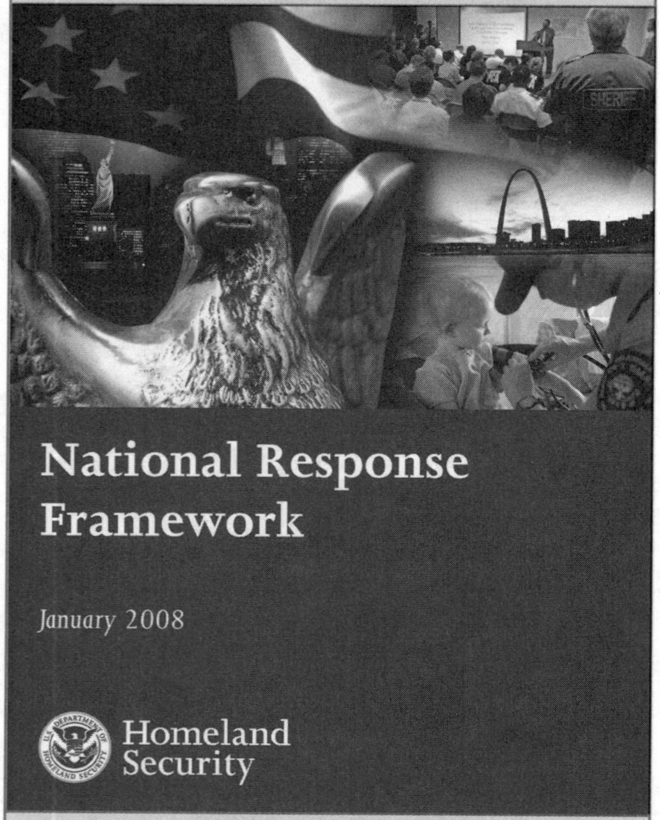

Source: Homeland Security http://www.fema.gov/pdf/emergency/nrf/nrf-core.pdf

BOX 5-3 Emergency Support Function 8 of the National Response Framework—Public Health and Medical Services Annex

Purpose

Emergency Support Function (ESF) 8—Public Health and Medical Services provides the mechanism for coordinated Federal assistance to supplement State, tribal, and local resources in response to a public health and medical disaster, potential or actual incidents requiring a coordinated Federal response, and/or during a developing potential health and medical emergency. The phrase "medical needs" is used throughout this annex. Public Health and Medical Services include responding to medical needs associated with mental health, behavioral health, and substance abuse considerations of incident victims and response workers. Services also cover the medical needs of members of the "at risk" or "special needs" population described in the Pandemic and All-Hazards Preparedness Act and in the *National Response Framework (NRF)* Glossary, respectively. It includes a population whose members may have medical and other functional needs before, during, and after an incident.

Public Health and Medical Services includes behavioral health needs consisting of both mental health and substance abuse considerations for incident victims and response workers and, as appropriate, medical needs groups defined in the core document as individuals in need of additional medical response assistance, and veterinary and/or animal health issues."

ESF Coordinator:

Department of Health and Human Services

Support Agencies:

Department of Agriculture

Department of Commerce

Department of Defense

Department of Energy

Department of Homeland Security

Department of the Interior

Department of Justice

Department of Labor

Department of State

Department of Transportation

Department of Veterans Affairs

Environmental Protection Agency

General Services Administration

U.S. Agency for International Development

U.S. Postal Service

American Red Cross

Primary Agency:

Department of Health and Human Services

Source: Emergency Support Function 8—Public Health and Medical Services Annex. National Response Framework. January 2008.

sponse are coordinated. These issues could include law enforcement needs, international implications of the outbreak, containing an epidemic, assessing any potential environmental contamination, and possible needs for decontamination procedures.

One of the most challenging questions posed by these guidance documents is Who is in charge? If a public health emergency turns out to be caused by an intentional event, then not only does the public health community need to respond, but the law enforcement community will be in charge of all legal and investigatory aspects. Because there may be both intelligence and foreign affairs equities at stake, those communities are brought into the fold as well. And the Department of Homeland Security remains tasked with coordinating communication with the public.

In all, NIMS and the NRF are designed to work together to better coordinate and prepare all entities that may be involved in responding to emergencies. NIMS is the "template for the management of incidents,"[7] while the NRF focuses on the mechanisms for policy and operational direction at the federal level.

PRESIDENTIAL POLICY DIRECTIVE 8

In March 2011, the Obama administration released Presidential Policy Directive 8—National Preparedness, replacing HSPD 8. The PPD calls for the development of a national preparedness goal (as did HSPD 8) and the creation of a National Preparedness System to integrate guidance programs and processes to build and sustain capabilities essential for preparedness. This directive takes an "all-of-Nation" approach, identifying the importance of collaboration between governments at all levels and the private and nonprofit sectors, as well as with the public, striving to enhance resilience.[8] Specifically, the directive defines resilience as "the ability to adapt to changing conditions and withstand and rapidly recover from disruption due to emergencies."[9] PPD 8 also calls for federal departments and agencies to develop operational planning frameworks, each with guidance to support state, local, and tribal government planning efforts.

STATE PREPAREDNESS

States have responsibility for developing their own emergency preparedness plans, and all have some level of planning and preparedness training in place. Preparedness efforts at the state level have strived to meet national preparedness objectives yet, at the same time, focus on the unique threats, challenges, assets, and populations specific to particular jurisdictions. States that are subject to hurricanes may have well developed plans to address that particular hazard, while landlocked states far from oceans may have better developed plans for disasters such as tornadoes. States will also take into account the particular demographics of their region when planning for vulnerable populations, nursing homes, and schools in emergencies. All states have more developed emer-

gency plans then pre-9/11, but all continue to have some gaps, be it around medical surge capacity, school-based preparedness, or preparedness for radiation events.[10,11,12]

The federal government has provided extensive funding to states to support preparedness planning and related activities. Between 2003 and 2007, DHS alone awarded over $27 billion in preparedness grants to state and local governments, although this represents only a small fraction of the total state and local preparedness expenditures.[13] In FY 2011, DHS allocated $2.1 billion for preparedness grants, although this represented a $780 million reduction from FY 2010.[14] Beyond funding, DHS also provides guidance. In November 2010, FEMA released an updated version of its *Comprehensive Preparedness Guide 101* to assist state and local entities in developing preparedness plans.[15]

DISCUSSION

This entire chapter begs the question, Does it work? Are we prepared? Is everyone ready for the next emergency? Will there be appropriate coordination of activities during the next emergency? The most honest answer is, probably, but we don't know. Planning and preparedness are a difficult balancing act. Funding is often associated with the previous disaster, in that monies are appropriated so we can better respond to the exact type of emergency that happened last time. Yet, seldom does the next emergency mirror the last. Scenario-based planning is useful but only as long as planners and responders are flexible enough to view these scenarios as illustrative of the potential set of capabilities that should be developed. A locality should not think it is fully prepared if it can check the box that it is ready for disaster A, B, and C. Because the next disaster will most certainly not match the planning scenarios. This means that the best we can do as a nation is to be as forward thinking as possible regarding potential emergencies so that we can enable a flexible and coordinated response, with appropriate resources, using the best possible risk communication methods.

KEY WORDS

National Response Framework
National Incident Management System
Preparedness planning
Exercise and evaluation
Presidential Policy Directive 8

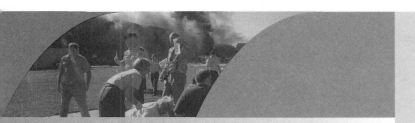

Discussion Questions

1. Describe current U.S. government policies regarding management of domestic emergencies.

2. What is the division among federal, state, and local entities in an emergency?

3. What documents answer the question, Who is in charge?

4. How is NIMS different from NRF? How do they work together?

5. Is it best to have national consistency in preparedness planning, or is it better to have plans that are specific to particular jurisdictions? Should there be a combination of both approaches?

6. How would you organize preparedness planning for federal, state, and local entities to best prepare for the next emergency?

REFERENCES

1. The White House. Homeland Security Presidential Directive 5: Management of Domestic Incidents. February 28, 2003. Available at: http://www.dhs.gov/xabout/laws/gc_1214592333605.shtm#1. Accessed August 23, 2010.

2. The White House. Homeland Security Directive 8: National Preparedness. December 17, 2003. Available at: http://www.dhs.gov/xabout/laws/gc_1215444247124.shtm. Accessed August 23, 2010.

3. U.S. Department of Homeland Security. *National Preparedness Guidelines*. September 2007. Available at: http://www.fema.gov/pdf/government/npg.pdf. Accessed August 23, 2010.

4. U.S. Department of Homeland Security. *National Response Framework*. January 2008. Available at: http://www.fema.gov/pdf/emergency/nrf/nrf-core.pdf. Accessed August 23, 2010.

5. Federal Emergency Management Agency. Emergency Support Function 8—Public Health and Medical Services Annex. January 2008. Available at: http://www.fema.gov/pdf/emergency/nrf/nrf-esf-08.pdf. Accessed August 23, 2010.

6. Federal Emergency Management Agency. Biological Incident Annex. August 2008. Available at: http://www.fema.gov/pdf/emergency/nrf/nrf_BiologicalIncidentAnnex.pdf. Accessed August 23, 2010.

7. U.S. Department of Homeland Security. About the National Incident Management System (NIMS). Available at: http://www.fema.gov/emergency/nims/AboutNIMS.shtm. Accessed August 23, 2010.

8. Balboni M, Kaniewski D, Paulison RD. Preparedness, Response and Resilience Task Force: Interim Task Force Report on Resilience. Homeland Security Policy Institute. May 16, 2011. Available at: http://www.gwumc.edu/hspi/policy/report_Resilience1.pdf. Accessed May 20, 2011.

9. The White House. *Presidential Policy Directive-8, National Preparedness*. March 30, 2011. Available at: http://www.dhs.gov/xabout/laws/gc_1215444247124.shtm. Accessed May 19, 2011.

10. Watkins WM, Perrotta D, Stanbury M, et al. State-level emergency preparedness and response capabilities. *Disaster Medicine and Public Health Preparedness*. 2011; 5:3134–3142.

11. GAO. Emergency Management: Most School Districts Have Developed Emergency Management Plans, but Would Benefit From Additional Federal Guidance. GAO-07-609. Washington DC. June 2007.

12. GAO. Emergency Preparedness: State Efforts to Plan for Medical Surge Could Benefit from Shared Guidance for Allocating Scarce Medical Resources. GAO-10-381T. Washington DC. January 25, 2010.

13. Local, State, Tribal and Federal Preparedness Task Force. Perspective on Preparedness: Taking Stock Since 9/11. Report to Congress. September 2010. Available at: http://www.fema.gov/pdf/preparednesstaskforce/perspective_on_preparedness.pdf. Accessed May 19, 2011.

14. Department of Homeland Security. DHS Announces Grant Guidance for Fiscal Year 2011 Preparedness Grants. May 19, 2011. Available at: http://www.dhs.gov/ynews/releases/pr_1305812474325.shtm. Accessed May 19, 2011.

15. Federal Emergency Management Agency. Developing and Maintaining Emergency Operations Plans: Comprehensive Preparedness Guide 101, Version 2.0. November 2010. Available at: http://www.fema.gov/pdf/about/divisions/npd/CPG_101_V2.pdf. Accessed May 19, 2011.

CHAPTER 6

Legislation, Regulations, and Policy Guidance

LEARNING OBJECTIVES

By the end of this chapter, the reader will be able to:

- Identify legislation, regulations, and policies that frame public health preparedness.
- Describe current policy positions on preparedness, particularly as they relate to biological threats.
- Understand the debate between security and civil liberties that arise from the Model State Emergency Health Powers Act.

INTRODUCTION

Legislation, regulations, and policy guidance documents form the foundation of public health preparedness. In other disciplines, these documents might be considered the "theory" that underlies the study. In this ever-evolving, operations-based field, it is the legal and regulatory framework that creates the baseline for which all policy, planning, and action is taken. As this is a relatively new discipline, the legislation, regulation, and policy guidance are also relatively new, changing to meet an evolving threat, incorporating lessons from previous experiences, and adapting to feedback from those directly affected by these documents. This chapter looks at a variety of public laws, regulations, and presidential directives that have shaped the field over the past decade. All legislation and executive orders related to select agents are addressed in the next chapter.

Previous chapters looked at guidance documents that support emergency and disaster preparedness and response. This included a review of the Stafford Act, which gives the president the power to issue major disaster declarations in response to emergencies that overwhelm state and local authorities. This chapter examines a series of laws and policy guidance that support preparedness efforts. We first look chronologically at a series of legislations and then explore presidential directives. Finally, we discuss a model piece of legislation and the debate it raises over the balance between individual rights and the powers needed to respond effectively to an emergency.

LEGISLATION

Public Health Improvement Act of 2000 (Public Law 106-505)

The Public Health Improvement Act of 2000 has 10 titles, or sections, 9 of which address traditional public health interests, such as sexually transmitted diseases, Alzheimer's research, organ donation, clinical research, and laboratory infrastructure. Title 1, however, addresses emerging threats to public health. This section authorizes the Secretary of Department of Health and Human Services (DHHS) to take appropriate response actions during a public health emergency, including investigations, treatment, and prevention. The act established the Public Health Emergency Fund to support activities in response to such public health emergencies. The act also authorized 10 years of appropriations to the CDC to defend and combat public health threats. Of note, the act directs the Secretary of DHHS to establish a working group to focus on the medical and public health effects of a bioterrorist attack.

USA Patriot Act of 2001 (Public Law 107-56)

The Uniting and Strengthening America by Providing Appropriate Tools Required to Intercept and Obstruct Terrorism (USA PATRIOT) Act passed in October 2001, immediately following the 9/11 attacks and during the height of the anthrax-letters scare. This act addressed a multitude of terrorism-related issues. In addition to provisions on select agents (which will be covered in the next chapter), the Patriot Act included assistance to first responders and indicated the desire of Congress for substantial new investments in bioterrorism preparedness and response.[1](§ 1013)

Public Health Security and Bioterrorism Preparedness and Response Act of 2002 (Public Law 107-188)

The June 2002 Bioterrorism Act was the first major piece of legislation dedicated entirely to public health preparedness. The act had five titles:

I. National Preparedness for Bioterrorism and Other Public Health Emergencies. This section addressed national preparedness and response planning by calling for the development and maintenance of medical countermeasures, creation of a national disaster medical system, support for communications and surveillance among all levels of public health officials, creation of a core curriculum for teaching about bioweapons and other public health emergencies, improving hospital preparedness, and addressing workforce shortages for public health emergencies.

   Interestingly, this title also codifies what had already been established—a strategic national stockpile of medical countermeasures. Specifically, the law directs DHHS to ensure that there is enough smallpox vaccine in the stockpile to "meet the health security needs of the United States." It also specifically calls for the stockpile to have enough potassium iodide tablets to distribute to populations within 20 miles of a nuclear power plant.[2](Title I, Subtitle B)

II. Enhancing Controls on Dangerous Biological Agents and Toxins. This title addresses the control over select agents.

III. Protecting Safety and Security of Food and Drug Supply. Title III is focused on bioterrorist threats to the food supply and outlines what the FDA is permitted to do to address this threat. It also touches on the importance of ensuring the safety of drugs imported into the United States.

IV. Drinking Water Security and Safety. This section of the law directs communities to do a full assessment of the vulnerabilities of the water supply to terrorist attacks.

V. Additional Provisions. This final section of the law includes provisions for prescription drug user fees, digital televisions, and Medicare plans.

Smallpox Emergency Personnel Protection Act of 2003 (Public Law 108-20)

The next piece of legislation passed after the Bioterrorism Act was the Smallpox Emergency Personnel Protection Act (SEPPA). In December 2002, the Bush administration announced a program to vaccinate both military personnel and civilian emergency health workers against smallpox. The vaccine program for the military was obligatory, while the civilian vaccination program was voluntary. This act, which became law almost 3 months after the vaccination program described in **Box 6-1** started, focuses on compensation related to medical care, lost income, or death resulting from the smallpox vaccine.

The Project Bioshield Act of 2004 (Public Law 108-276)

While the Bioterrorism Act of 2002 codified the Strategic National Stockpile, there was a problem getting the pharmaceutical industry to invest in creating medical countermeasures (drugs and vaccines) to address the CBRN threat, thus creating a lack of medical tools in the stockpile. Because of the vast costs involved, pharmaceutical companies were reluctant to start the process of developing and bringing to market CBRN medical countermeasures without a guaranteed market. The Bioshield Act of 2004 aimed to create a guaranteed, government-funded market for these countermeasures and funding to purchase the products while they are still in the final stages of development. The act also allowed DHHS to expedite spending to procure products, hire experts, and award research grants pertaining to CBRN and to allow for emergency use of countermeasures even if they lack final FDA approval.

Public Readiness and Emergency Preparedness (PREP) Act of 2005 (Division C of the Department of Defense Emergency Supplemental Appropriations, Public Law 109-148)

The purpose of the PREP Act was to limit liability associated with public health countermeasures used on an emer-

BOX 6-1 2003 Smallpox Vaccination Program

On December 13, 2002, President George W. Bush announced a plan to vaccinate military and select civilian personnel against smallpox, citing national security concerns. These concerns were based on general fears of a bioterrorism attack against the United States using smallpox, a disease that has been eradicated and for which the general population had little to no immunity. The United States ceased routine vaccination of smallpox in 1972, and even for those who had been vaccinated prior, immunity had diminished significantly.

The administration's plan was to vaccinate 500,000 military personnel against smallpox as fast as possible and then vaccinate 500,000 civilians, focusing first on healthcare workers and first responders. Initially, the debate among the civilian community was around who would be eligible, with multiple entities pushing for inclusion. When the time came to be vaccinated, however, far fewer civilians than expected participated. By January 2004, 578,286 military personnel were vaccinated, but only 34,213 civilians received the vaccine.

Many of the civilian health workers refused the vaccine, often citing the potential for adverse reactions because the vaccine is a live virus that has the potential to cause severe side effects. In fact, two civilians and one military member (all in their 50s) died within days of receiving the smallpox vaccine from ischemic cardiac events (heart attacks). Approximately 20 additional vaccine recipients suffered nonfatal cardiac events.

The National Academies of Science (NAS) found the smallpox vaccination program to have several major flaws contributing to its overall failure within the civilian population. NAS found that the rationale for the smallpox vaccination program was never clearly explained to key constituencies, the program assumptions were never reviewed, and CDC was constrained in its ability to communicate effectively to state and local public health officials. There were significant barriers to program implementation, such as lack of compensation at the start of the program, logistical and practical constraints, and confusion over program structure and goals. Additionally, the program did not explicitly link to preparedness, leaving stakeholders with questions about the utility of the program. NAS recommended that future preparedness programs better integrate public health and scientific reason, engage stakeholders, and establish strong communication lines to the public about preparedness efforts.

Sources: Richards EP, Rathbun KC, Gold J. The Smallpox Vaccination Campaign of 2003: Why did it fail and what are the lessons for bioterrorism preparedness? *Louisiana Law Review.* 2004;64:851–904; Available at: http://biotech.law.lsu.edu/articles/smallpox.pdf; Thaul S. *CRS Report for Congress: Smallpox Vaccine Injury Compensation.* The University of Maryland School of Law. June 13, 2003. Available at: http://www.law.umaryland.edu/marshall/crsreports/crsdocuments/RL31960.pdf. Accessed September 10, 2010; Centers for Disease Control and Prevention. Cardiac deaths after a mass smallpox vaccination campaign—New York City, 1947. *Morbidity and Mortality Weekly.* October 2003;52(39):933–936; Centers for Disease Control and Prevention. Update: Cardiac-related events during the civilian smallpox vaccination program—United States, 2003. *Morbidity and Mortality Weekly.* May 2003;52(21):492–496; and Committee on Smallpox Vaccination Program Implementation, Board on Health Promotion and Disease Prevention, Institute of Medicine. *The Smallpox Vaccination Program, Public Health in an Age of Terrorism.* Washington, DC: The National Academies Press; 2005, p. 5.

gency basis. The Project Bioshield Act allowed the secretary of DHHS to use medical countermeasures for emergency purposes without final FDA approval. This act ensures that manufacturers whose medical countermeasures are used without this final FDA approval—as well as distributors, program administrators, prescribers, or dispensers in this situation—cannot be sued if there are negative consequences associated with the use of the drug or vaccine. The only exception is in the event of "willful misconduct."

Pandemic and All-Hazards Preparedness Act of 2006 (Public Law 109-417)

This act, known as PAHPA, officially reauthorized the Bioterrorism Act of 2002 and included broad provisions aimed at preparing for and responding to public health and medical

emergencies regardless of origin. The act is organized into the following four main titles:

I. National Preparedness and Response, Leadership, Organization, and Planning. This title gives the secretary of DHHS the lead for all public health and medical responses to emergencies covered by the National Response Framework* (see Chapter 5). It also establishes the position of the assistant secretary for preparedness and response at DHHS and defines the purpose of this position for

---

* The act actually refers to the National Response Plan, which was later updated and renamed the National Response Framework.

public health and medical preparedness and response. In addition to specific preparedness activities, this title requires DHHS to create a National Health Security Strategy (see Chapter 3).

II. Public Health Security Preparedness. This section of the act focuses on developing preparedness infrastructure, primarily at the state and local levels, to include pandemic plans, interoperable networks for data sharing, and telehealth capabilities. This section also addresses laboratory security and the need to ensure readiness of the Commissioned Corps of the Public Health Service to respond to public health emergencies.

III. All-Hazards Medical Surge Capacity. This title has several major provisions, including the transfer of the National Disaster Medical System (NDMS) back to DHHS from DHS. DHHS is responsible for evaluating capacity for a surge during a public health emergency and is required to establish a Medical Reserve Corps of volunteers to assist during such emergencies. Of interest, this title also requires DHHS to develop public health preparedness curricula (see Chapter 1) and establish centers for preparedness at schools of public health.

IV. Pandemic and Biodefense Vaccine and Drug Development. This final title of the act builds off of the Bioshield Act of 2004 and calls for the establishment of the Biomedical Advanced Research and Development Authority (BARDA) within DHHS to coordinate countermeasure research and development. Although the Bioshield Act helped entice manufacturers to develop countermeasures, it did not do enough to get companies through the expensive years of research and development. This title allows BARDA to change the payment structure to better enable countermeasure development and production.

Implementing Recommendations of the 9/11 Commission Act of 2007 (Public Law 110-53)

In August 2007, Congress passed the Implementing Recommendations of the 9/11 Commission Act, which as the title suggests, focuses on implementing the recommendations from the *9/11 Commission Report*. The act focuses on numerous specific provisions pertaining to preparedness, such as preparedness grants to state and local entities, improving the incident command system, improving the sharing of intelligence information across the federal government, enhancing efforts to prevent terrorists from traveling to the United States, safety of transportation, and basic overall improvements to the preparedness infrastructure. It also includes sections on advancing democratic values abroad and diplomatic engagement. Specific to public health, Title XI of the act addresses enhanced defense against weapons of mass destruction and specifically focuses on the need to maintain a National Biosurveillance Integration Center and report to Congress on the "state of . . . biosurveillance efforts."[3(§ 1102)]

PENDING LEGISLATION

In addition to the preceding legislation, other legislation has been introduced in Congress over the years pertaining to public health preparedness, but none has ever become law. The Pathogen Security Act, which addressed global surveillance and capacity building around dangerous pathogens, was introduced several times over the last decade although it never made it out of the Senate. The WMD Prevention and Preparedness Act of 2009 built on the Pathogen Security Act, but at the time of this writing, it has not progressed to a Senate vote. It may, however, be re-introduced in late 2011. Several additional bills have been proposed, all trying to address surveillance, training, and security associated with infectious diseases and bioterrorism. None of these bills, however, has had much traction. This is not necessarily due to any fatal flaws in the proposed legislation but rather a combination of the immediacy of the threat, other pressing issues in Congress, the timing of the bills' introductions, the abundance of other legislation addressing similar themes, and the work already being conducted by the federal agencies without legislative support.

PAHPA expires soon, and we should expect to see a reauthorization bill passed by the end of 2011.

PRESIDENTIAL DIRECTIVES

In previous chapters, we looked at presidential directives, primarily as they applied to creating the preparedness infrastructure (e.g., HSPD 5 and 8 and PPD 8). Here, we examine five more presidential directives that helped form the policy guidance and regulations for public health preparedness.

Biodefense for the 21st Century (National Security Presidential Directive 33/Homeland Security Presidential Directive 10, April 2004)

In 2004, the Bush administration released Biodefense for the 21st Century (HSPD 10), which provided a strategic overview of the biological threat and the way to frame biodefense initiatives. The directive described four essential pillars of the national biodefense program: threat awareness, prevention and protection, surveillance and detection, and response and recovery. This document would remain the primary policy directive for biodefense until the National Strategy for Countering Biological Threats was released in late 2009.

Medical Countermeasures Against Weapons of Mass Destruction (Homeland Security Presidential Directive 18, February 2007)

Following HSPD 10, the Bush administration released HSPD 18 on the development of medical countermeasures to counter WMDs. The directive defined the policies associated with medical countermeasures—from focused development of agent-specific countermeasures to a flexible capability for future countermeasures. DHHS was directed to lead research, development, evaluation, and acquisition of public health emergency medical countermeasures, while DoD retained control over countermeasure development specifically for the armed forces.

Public Health and Medical Preparedness (Homeland Security Presidential Directive 21, October 2007)

Building upon HSPD 10 and in accordance with HSPD 18, HSPD 21 was released in the fall of 2007 and defines four critical components of public health and medical preparedness: a robust and integrated biosurveillance system, the ability to stockpile and distribute medical countermeasures, capacity to engage in mass casualty care in emergency situations, and building resilient communities at the state and local levels. In addition to identifying these critical areas, the directive mandates the creation of task forces, studies, and plans to meet public health and medical preparedness needs. There are also calls for implementation of aspects of PAHPA, including the development of core curricula in preparedness and the inclusion of the principles outlined in the directive in the National Health Security Strategy.

Establishing Federal Capability for the Timely Provision of Medical Countermeasures Following a Biological Attack (Executive Order 13527, December 2009)

In the last days of 2009, Executive Order 13527 was released, establishing a policy of timely provision of medical countermeasures in the event of a biological attack and tasking the federal government with assisting state and local entities in this endeavor. This EO also spells out the role of the United States Postal Service (USPS) for delivery of medical counter-measures. (See **Box 6-2.**) This order also calls for DHHS to develop continuity of operations plans in the event of a large-scale biological attack.

National Strategy for Countering Biological Threats (Presidential Policy Directive 2, November 2009)

The National Strategy for Countering Biological Threats was released in time for Under Secretary of State Ellen Tauscher to share it with the international community at the December 2009 Meeting of States Parties of the Biological Weapons Convention.[4] The strategy, the first major policy statement by the Obama administration on biological threats, describes the spectrum of biological threats and then spells out seven major objectives (spelling out PROTECT):

> **Promote** global health security;
>
> **Reinforce** norms of safe and responsible conduct;
>
> **Obtain** timely and accurate insight on current and emerging risks;
>
> **Take** reasonable steps to reduce the potential for exploitation;

BOX 6-2 United States Postal Service as Distributor of Medical Countermeasures

In 2001, the United States Postal Service became an overnight stakeholder in biodefense when mail sorters and carriers became exposed to anthrax, as the agent was delivered through letters to key targets. Not only did some postal workers become exposed, but several became ill, and two employees of the Brentwood mail facility in Washington, DC, died.

Several years after the anthrax letters, the Postal Service was identified as the best means of rapid residential delivery of medical countermeasures following a biological attack. In late 2009, the Obama administration released an executive order stating the government would develop models for postal service response to large-scale emergencies, where medical countermeasures would need to be delivered to large populations in a short period of time. As part of this postal plan, USPS, with accompanying law enforcement support, will deliver medication to each household, with information sheets regarding how and when to take the medication.

Expand our capability to prevent, attribute, and apprehend;

Communicate effectively with all stakeholders; and

Transform the international dialogue on biological threats.[5,6]

While many of the Bush administration's directives focused on policies to respond to a biological threat, this strategy puts more emphasis on prevention, with particular stress on the importance of working with international partners, reinforcing norms of responsible scientific conduct, and engaging scientists so that they can continue beneficial work in the life sciences while being cognizant of potential threats.

MODEL LEGISLATION

During a public health emergency, it is essential to have legal authorities in place that allow the government to mount an effective response, mitigate the consequences of the event, and save lives. Public health authority is primarily a power left to the state and local governments,[7(Amend. X)] but many states do not have appropriate legislation in place to effectively deal with a public health crisis. In fact, some states have public health laws that are inconsistent, complicated, and often outdated.[8] With the shift in thinking regarding public health emergencies as potential national security concerns, legal experts embarked on an exercise to provide model legislation to enable states to revisit their legislative toolkit. In December 2001, Professor Lawrence Gostin, funded by the Centers for Disease Control and Prevention, released the Model State Emergency Health Powers Act (MSEHPA).[9]

The MSEHPA was designed to allow state and local health authorities to effectively respond to public health emergencies and is structured into five basic public health functions:

1. Preparedness.
2. Surveillance.
3. Management of property.
4. Protection of persons (including compelling vaccination, treatment, isolation, and quarantine).
5. Communication.

The model law tries to balance the need to provide state and local authorities with the ability to manage a public health emergency with the need to protect civil liberties and safeguard personal rights. The model law prompted much debate about the role of the federal government in responding to emergencies versus state responsibilities, the fear of abuse of power, personal and economic liberties during an emergency, and safeguarding of property. It also brought strong opposition from individuals and groups not comfortable with a government entity forcing vaccination, medical examination, quarantine, rapid burials, and takeover of private property—even if in response to an emergency. Some felt this was too much of an affront to civil liberties and not worth the sacrifice for the common good. Others were concerned that such powers might be abused by government authorities and applied in nonemergency situations.

This act has been introduced in whole or in part in more than 170 bills in 44 states, and 38 states have passed bills or resolutions that contain provisions from the model law.

SUMMARY

Legislation and regulations form an essential foundation to public health emergency preparedness, and much has been done in the past decade to solidify this foundation. Many of these rules, however, are continually revisited and will no doubt evolve over the next few years as the nation improves its overall preparedness activities.

KEY WORDS

Legislation
Presidential directives
National strategy
Pandemic and All Hazards Preparedness Act
Model legislation

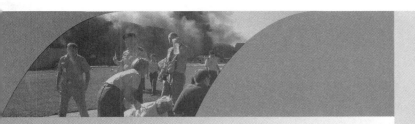

Discussion Questions

1. How do legislation and regulations support public health preparedness?

2. What would happen if these laws were not in place?

3. What is missing in the legal landscape of public health preparedness?

4. Is there one particular law, regulation, or directive that you think is most important? Why?

5. How would you balance civil liberties and common good during a public health emergency?

REFERENCES

1. Uniting and Strengthening America by Providing Appropriate Tools Required to Intercept and Obstruct Terrorism (USA PATRIOT) Act of 2001; Public Law No. 107-56.

2. Public Health Security and Bioterrorism Preparedness and Response Act of 2002; Public Law No. 107-188.

3. Implementing Recommendations of the 9/11 Commission Act of 2007; Public Law No. 110-53.

4. Under Secretary of State Ellen O. Tauscher. Address to States Parties of the BWC. *United States Mission to the United Nations and Other International Organizations in Geneva*. December 9, 2009. Available at: http://geneva.usmission.gov/2009/12/09/tauscher-bwc/. Accessed September 10, 2010.

5. National Security Council. *National Strategy for Countering Biological Threats*. November 2009. Available at: http://www.whitehouse.gov/sites/default/files/National_Strategy_for_Countering_BioThreats.pdf. Accessed September 10, 2010.

6. Miller JE. National Strategy for Countering Biological Threats. In: Katz R, Zilinikas R, eds. *Encyclopedia of Bioterrorism Defense*, 2nd ed. Wiley and Sons; May 2011.

7. Constitution of the United States of America.

8. Hodge JJG, Gostin LO, Gebbie K, Erickson DL. Transforming Public Health Law: The Turning Point Model State Public Health Act. *Journal of Law, Medicine & Ethics*. Spring 2006;34(1):77–84.

9. Gostin LO. The Model State Emergency Health Powers Act. *The Centers for Law & the Public's Health*. December 21, 2001. Available at: http://www.publichealthlaw.net/MSEHPA/MSEHPA.pdf. Accessed September 10, 2010.

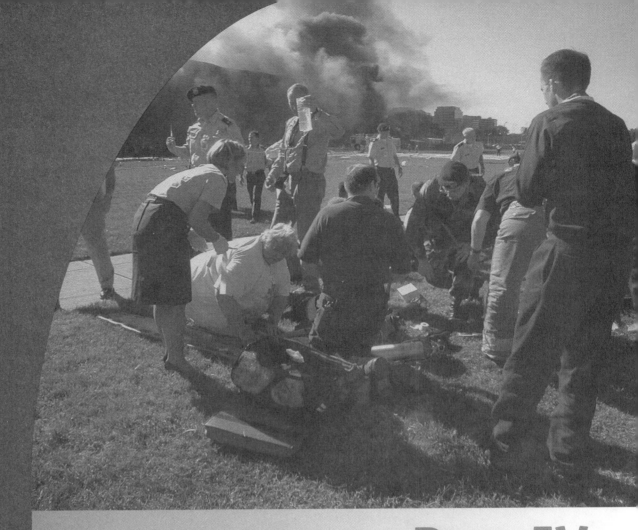

PART IV

Solving Problems

CHAPTER 7

Biosecurity

LEARNING OBJECTIVES

By the end of this chapter, the reader will be able to:

- Define biosecurity.
- Describe how biosecurity is used to minimize biological threats.
- Discuss the dual-use dilemma.
- Describe the policy positions and guidance that have evolved around scientific research, publications, and the control of select agents.
- Understand the purpose, past and future, of the cooperative threat reduction programs.
- Assess the threat posed by synthetic biology.

INTRODUCTION

In previous chapters, we looked at the public health threats from both weapons of mass destruction and naturally occurring disease. We have examined the infrastructure and legislative and regulatory environments that have evolved over the past decade that support public health preparedness. In this next section of the book, we start to look at how some of the challenges and threats are being addressed in an attempt to "solve problems." This chapter will examine biosecurity and biosafety; discuss the dual-use dilemma in scientific research; and describe the policy positions and guidance that have evolved around research, publications, and the control of dangerous pathogens. We will also look at some of the programs adopted by the U.S. government to reduce the threat posed by weapons of mass destruction.

Biosecurity is a process to reduce or eliminate the ability of a biological agent to adversely affect human, animal,

or plant health, as well as the economy or the environment. It is the management of biological and environmental risks, whether the risks come from the agents themselves, infectious diseases, invasive species, or biological weapons. Biosecurity is also the protection of agents or facilities "against the theft or diversion of high-consequence microbial agents, which could be used by someone who maliciously intends to conduct bioterrorism or pursue biological weapons proliferation."[1(p 7)] Achieving biosecurity, or in the case of protection of agents, pathogen security, involves physically protecting agents (i.e., locking them up, securing facilities); ensuring the staff working with these agents take responsibility for the safety and security of the agents themselves; and implementing other administrative measures to enhance accountability, security, and oversight.

Biosafety, often mistakenly used interchangeably with *biosecurity* (and in some languages they are the same word), is the process used to prevent people and the environment from being exposed to hazardous biological agents. Biosafety is about safely handling infectious agents through the application of proper techniques, equipment, and personal behavior, as demonstrated in **Table 7-1**, which explains the different biosafety levels. The simple phrase used to distinguish biosafety from biosecurity is "Biosafety is about protecting people from bad bugs; biosecurity is about protecting bugs from bad people."[2(p 27)]

Biorisk is the name given to the chance that any type of adverse event leading to potential harm will occur—be it an accidental infection within the laboratory or the loss, theft, unauthorized access, or intentional release of an agent.[3] Biorisk management, then, is the development of strategies

TABLE 7-1 Biosafety Levels (BSL) for Infectious Agents

Depending on the type of agent one is working with, there are recommended biosafety measures that should be taken. These measures range from best practices by the laboratorian, to the infrastructure necessary to work safely with agents. There are four biosafety levels that prescribe how to work with increasingly dangerous infectious agents. The table below is derived from the *Biosafety in Microbiological and Biomedical Laboratories* (*BMBL*), 5th Edition.

BSL	Agents	Equipment and Facilities for Appropriate Barriers
1	Do not usually lead to disease in healthy adults. (Example: nonpathogenic *E. coli*	Lab coats and gloves Face and eye protection as needed Laboratory bench and sink
2	Agents cause disease but not through inhalation. (Example: HIV or *Yersinia pestis*)	Lab coats and gloves Face and eye protection as needed Physical containment devices for manipulations of agents that cause splashes or aerosols of agents BSL 1 facilities + Autoclave
3	Agents that cause serious or potentially lethal disease through inhalation. (Example: Tuberculosis or St. Louis encephalitis)	Protective lab clothing and gloves Face, eye, and respiratory protection as needed Physical containment devices for all open manipulations of agents BSL 2 facilities + physical separation from access corridors, double-door access, negative airflow, entry through airlock or anteroom, handwashing sink near lab exit
4	Dangerous or exotic agents that are frequently fatal and for which there are no vaccines or treatments. These agents may have an unknown risk of transmission or have a high risk of aerosol transmission. (Example: Ebola)	All primary barriers, equipment, and procedures conducted in BSL 3 or procedures conducted with equipment from BSLs 1 and 2 in combination with a full-body, air-supplied, positive pressure suit BSL 3 facilities + separate building or isolated areas, dedicated supply and exhaust, vacuum and decontamination system, and other specified safety requirements

Source: Centers for Disease Control and Prevention. Section IV—Laboratory Biosafety Level Criteria. Biosafety in Microbiological and Biomedical Laboratories, 5th Edition.

incorporating both biosafety and biosecurity techniques to minimize the occurrences of biorisks and to manage the consequences. This integrated approach to biological threats within the laboratory environment is the responsibility of individual laboratories.[3]

The technical aspects of biosafety are outside the purview of this text, but we focus here on biosecurity, the problems for science posed by the dual-use dilemma, the debate over codes of conduct for life science researchers and efforts to regulate biosecurity.

THE DUAL-USE DILEMMA

Within the life sciences, "dual use" refers to research, agents, technologies, equipment, or information that can be used both for legitimate scientific purposes and for malevolent use to threaten public health or security.[4] The U.S. National Sci-

ence Advisory Board for Biosecurity (NSABB) defined dual-use research of concern as specifically "Research that, based on current understanding, can be reasonably anticipated to provide knowledge, products, or technologies that could be directly misapplied by others to pose a threat to public health and safety agricultural crops and other plants, animals, the environment, or materiel."[5(p 2)]

Life science research, particularly biological research, is grounded in the idea that research is good; it advances science and, thus, mankind; it saves lives; and in order to grow and develop, there must be open communication among researchers. This openness, however, becomes complicated when security is at risk. Scientists and security experts have struggled for decades to determine the right balance to ensure advances in life sciences while being aware of and mitigating the threat posed by the same research. This tension goes back to the 1940s in the post–World War II society. The 1947 President's Scientific Research Board report on Science and Public Policy wrote, "However important secrecy about military weapons may be, the fundamental discoveries of researchers must circulate freely to have full beneficial effect. ... Security regulations, therefore, should be applied only when strictly necessary."[6,7] This concept was echoed by President Harry Truman in 1948, when he said, "Continuous research by our best scientists is the key to American scientific leadership and true national security."[8] This position, although not always easy—particularly in physics, where technology was being used to make nuclear weapons and other weapons systems—remained the position of the government and researchers alike. This sentiment, however, began to change in the 1980s at the height of the Cold War. Advanced technology was acquired from U.S. universities and the government national laboratories by adversarial nations.[9] In 1980, the National Academies suspended its bilateral exchanges.[10(p 31)] In 1982, Executive Order 12356 broadened authorities to classify information but reiterated that "basic scientific research information not clearly related to national security may not be classified."[11] The same year, the National Academy of Sciences was asked to examine whether scientific information needed to be controlled. The subsequent report, *Scientific Communication and National Security*, also known as the Corson Report, had several major findings: that security by secrecy would weaken the United States; that there is no practical way to restrict international scientific communication; and that, while there has been a significant transfer of scientific information from the United States to adversarial countries, transfers of information from universities and through the publication of fundamental research were very small.[12]

In 1985, the Reagan administration released National Security Decision Directive (NSDD) 189. This directive stated, "It is the policy of this Administration that, to the maximum extent possible, the products of fundamental research remain unrestricted ... that, where the national security requires control, the mechanism for control of information generated during federally-funded fundamental research in science, technology and engineering at colleges, universities and laboratories is classification."[13] The responsibility for classification of research was given to the federal governmental agencies that supported the research (including external grants to researchers), and no restrictions were allowed on the conduct or reporting of the research that did not receive a national security classification.[13]

This policy from 1985 was reiterated right after September 11, 2001. In a letter from Dr. Condoleeza Rice, then National Security Advisor, and reaffirmed by Dr. John Mar-burger, science advisor, in congressional testimony,[14] the administration confirmed that "the policy on the transfer of scientific, technical, and engineering information set forth in NSDD-189 shall remain in effect, and we will ensure that this policy is followed."[15]

Mousepox

In 2001, a team of Australian researchers inserted the gene for interleukin-4 (IL-4) into the mousepox virus. The purpose of the study was to try to alter the virus so that it would make mice infertile and thus become a pest control method. They found that the recombinant virus killed mice genetically resistant to mousepox, as well as mice that had been immunized. When the researchers published their findings,[16] scientists around the world voiced concerns that the researchers had published a road map for increasing the lethality of mousepox by showing how to kill mice even after they had been immunized and, by extension, demonstrating how to increase the lethality of smallpox. Critics quickly claimed that the article should never have been published and that this "dual-use" research could easily be picked up by terrorists and used to make a biological weapon that would circumvent our medical countermeasures.[17]

The publication of this mousepox experiment raised a series of questions for the scientific community. Should the experiment have been done in the first place if researchers recognized the possible implications of the research? Should the research have been publicized given the findings? Should any journal have published it? These questions went beyond this particular experiment to the larger problem being posed for science. Other articles were published that sparked similar concerns.[18,19] The community had to decide if scientists should be constrained as to the research questions they could ask. Scientific journals had to determine their responsibility for publishing manuscripts with potentially sensitive information. And, the security community in the United States began to question the number of foreign students and scholars being trained and working in domestic universities and research environments.

In 2003, the journal editors responded. (See **Box 7-1**.) Thirty-two largely American-based scientific journals agreed to guidelines for reviewing, modifying, and even rejecting research articles where the potential harm of publication might outweigh the potential for societal benefits.[20]

The Fink Report

The same year, the National Academies published *Biotechnology Research in an Age of Terrorism*, also known as the Fink Report (**Figure 7-1**). The purpose of the Fink Report was to

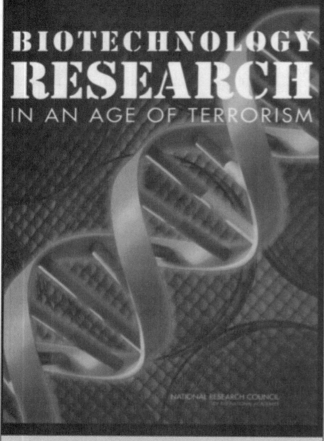

FIGURE 7-1 Biotechnology Research in an Age of Terrorism

Source: Committee on Research Standards and Practices to Prevent the Destructive Application of Biotechnology, National Research Council. Biotechnology Research in an Age of Terrorism. Reprinted with permission from the National Academies Press, Copyright 2004, National Academy of Sciences.

Biodefense to provide advice, guidance, and leadership on whether research should be published. The report identified seven types of "experiments of concern" that should be evaluated. The question posed was whether proceeding with the experiment would:

1. Render a vaccine to a pathogen ineffective.
2. Confer antibiotic resistance to a pathogen so as to decrease the effectiveness of a countermeasure.
3. Increase the virulence of a pathogen.
4. Increase the transmissibility of a pathogen.
5. Increase the host range/tropism of a pathogen.
6. Enable evasion of diagnostic/detection capabilities.
7. Demonstrate weaponization of a pathogen.

If an experiment met any of these criteria, it would require review. The government took these recommendations seriously and created what is known as the National Science Advisory Board for Biosecurity (NSABB). NSABB is an advisory board to the Secretary of Health and Human Services made up of scientists and ex-officio members from across the federal government. In addition to recommendations on criteria for identifying dual-use research of concern, NSABB provides national guidelines for oversight of dual-use research and advises on educational programs, codes of conduct for scientists, guidelines for dissemination of research methodologies and results, and strategies for international dialogues on dual-use research.

To date, two articles have been submitted to NSABB for review. The first was the complete genetic sequencing of the 1918 influenza virus. Some argued that the data were important for better understanding of flu and thus enabled current researchers to more adequately prepare for a future pandemic.[21] Others argued that "The genome is essentially the design of a weapon of mass destruction" and should not have been published.[22]

Another controversial article that provided a detailed description of how to contaminate the milk supply with Botulinum toxin was published by the Proceedings of the National Academies of Science (PNAS).[23] The authors argued that the paper was a wake-up call to enhance preparedness activities. Critics, however, saw it as a road map for bioterrorism. The paper was initially published online by PNAS but then pulled for review by NSABB. When it was finally published in the journal, some details had been removed from the article to make it less of a "how-to" for terrorists.

Today, we still do not really know how best to handle the dangerous aspects of science. At the same time, we do not want to constrain scientific advancement. Much of the current discussion is around setting up voluntary "codes of

develop a system to help reduce the threat of misuse of the life sciences, while protecting scientific research and communication to the maximum extent possible. The report proposed a system, based mostly on voluntary self-governance by the scientific community, that would have experiments reviewed at several stages to evaluate for dual-use concerns. The proposed system of review included a review at the university level through an Institutional Biosafety Committee (IBC), followed by review at NIH (assuming NIH supported the research) through the NIH Recombinant Advisory Committee. The research would then be evaluated by the journal editors, followed by a proposed National Science Advisory Board for

BOX 7-1 Statement on Scientific Publication and Security by Journal Editors

Preamble

The process of scientific publication, through which new findings are reviewed for quality and then presented to the rest of the scientific community and the public, is a vital element in our national life. New discoveries reported in research papers have helped improve the human condition in myriad ways: protecting public health, multiplying agricultural yields, fostering technological development and economic growth, and enhancing global stability and security.

But new science, as we know, may sometimes have costs as well as benefits. The prospect that weapons of mass destruction might find their way into the hands of terrorists did not suddenly appear on September 11, 2001. A policy focus on nuclear proliferation, no stranger to the physics community, has been with us for many years. But the events of September 11 brought a new understanding of the urgency of dealing with terrorism. And the subsequent harmful use of infectious agents brought a new set of issues to the life sciences. As a result, questions have been asked by the scientists themselves and by some political leaders about the possibility that new information published in research journals might give aid to those with malevolent ends.

Journals that dealt especially with microbiology, infectious agents, public health, and plant and agricultural systems faced these issues earlier than some others, and have attempted to deal with them. The American Society of Microbiology, in particular, urged the National Academy of Sciences to take an active role in organizing a meeting of publishers, scientists, security experts, and government officials to explore the issues and discuss what steps might be taken to resolve them. In a one-day workshop at the Academy in Washington on January 9, 2003, an open forum was held for that purpose. A day later, a group of journal editors, augmented by scientist-authors, government officials, and others, held a separate meeting designed to explore possible approaches.

What follows reflects some outcomes of that preliminary discussion. Fundamental is a view, shared by nearly all, that there is information that, although we cannot now capture it with lists or definitions, presents enough risk of use by terrorists that it should not be published. How and by what processes it might be identified will continue to challenge us, because—as all present acknowledged—it is also true that open publication brings benefits not only to public health but also to efforts to combat terrorism.

The Statements Follow:

FIRST: The scientific information published in peer-reviewed research journals carries special status, and confers unique responsibilities on editors and authors. We must protect the integrity of the scientific process by publishing manuscripts of high quality, in sufficient detail to permit reproducibility. Without independent verification—a requirement for scientific progress—we can neither advance biomedical research nor provide the knowledge base for building a strong biodefense system.

SECOND: We recognize that the prospect of bioterrorism has raised legitimate concerns about the potential abuse of published information, but also recognize that research in the very same fields will be critical to society in meeting the challenges of defense. We are committed to dealing responsibly and effectively with safety and security issues that may be raised by papers submitted for publication, and to increasing our capacity to identify such issues as they arise.

THIRD: Scientists and their journals should consider the appropriate level and design of processes to accomplish effective review of papers that raise such security issues. Journals in disciplines that have attracted numbers of such papers have already devised procedures that might be employed as models in considering process design. Some of us represent some of those journals; others among us are committed to the timely implementation of such processes, about which we will notify our readers and authors.

FOURTH: We recognize that on occasion an editor may conclude that the potential harm of publication outweighs the potential societal benefits. Under such circumstances, the paper should be modified, or not be published. Scientific information is also communicated by other means: seminars, meetings, electronic posting, etc. Journals and scientific societies can play an important role in encouraging investigators to communicate results of research in ways that maximize public benefits and minimize risks of misuse.

Source: Reproduced from Statement on scientific publication and security. *Science*. February 2003; 229(5610):1149.

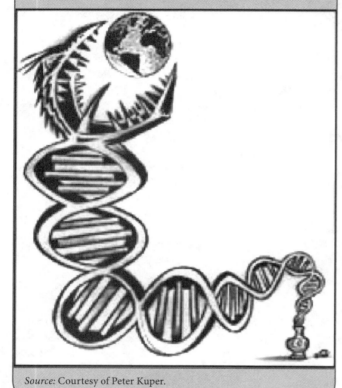

FIGURE 7-2 Germ Warfare. Political Cartoon from the *New York Times*. DNA Sequence Released Like a Genie in a Bottle to Threaten the Globe

Source: Courtesy of Peter Kuper.

conduct" for scientists to follow, giving them self-policing power to ensure the science they produce cannot be used for malevolent purposes. There is discussion about making this a part of the Responsible Conduct of Research—ethical guidelines for life science researchers.[24] The debate, though, continues to be waged regarding whether the control of dual-use research is a personal-level decision, a disciplinewide commitment, or a situation requiring government regulation or legal frameworks.

SELECT AGENTS

Since 1996, the government has tried to legislate how to handle potentially dangerous pathogens so they do not fall into the hands of people wishing to do harm. The first such legislation was the Antiterrorism and Effective Death Penalty Act of 1996.[25] The Act identified certain biological agents as posing a threat to society and provided that the transfer and possession of such agents should be regulated to protect public health and safety so only those with legitimate purposes would have access to the agents.[25(§ 511)] DHHS was to establish a list

of "select agents" for regulation, including those agents that cause significant morbidity and mortality, are contagious, or may not have medical countermeasures available. The authority to regulate the select agents was delegated to CDC, and CDC then required any laboratory transferring select agents to register and report any transfer.[26] In 1997, the select agent list had 42 biological agents and toxins.

The USA PATRIOT Act of 2001[27] furthered the 1996 law so that it became an offense to possess select biological agents or toxins without reasonable justification. The act also restricted possession or transfer of select agents to only approved individuals.

The Bioterrorism Act of 2002 added additional requirements for the possession or transfer of select agents, including requiring a background check by the FBI. This act also made regulation of the select agents a shared responsibility among CDC, USDA, and FBI. CDC is in charge of regulating human pathogens, while USDA has the lead for animal and plant pathogens. FBI leads any criminal investigative actions.

In July 2010, the Obama administration released Executive Order 13546 for Optimizing the Security of Biological Select Agents and Toxins in the United States.[28] The EO called for several things:

1. Tiering and the potential reduction of the select agent list: DHHS and USDA will tier the list of select agents to separate out those agents that require the most stringent physical security and personnel reliability measures so that other, less dangerous agents can have fewer restrictions. They will change the regulations accordingly.
2. Creation of a security advisory panel made up of federal experts: this panel will help with the tiering or reduction of the select agent list, as well as best practices for physical security and personnel reliability.

The overall body of laws and regulations on select agents makes it difficult to acquire and work with certain agents. It also makes clear that there are responsibilities that come with working with such agents. The effort to tier the agents is an attempt to retain the strictest regulations for the most dangerous agents but to ease up on other agents so that it is easier for researchers to conduct their work. The nature of research, however, has forever changed, and scientists must now take responsibility for the agents they work with. This shift can been seen in the case of Thomas Butler, described in **Box 7-2**.

SYNTHETIC BIOLOGY

Another area of concern for biosecurity is synthetic biology. This refers to the design and creation of biological components

BOX 7-2 The Case of Thomas Butler

Thomas Butler, 60, was a nationally recognized scientist at Texas Tech University Health Sciences Center in Lubbock for 15 years. After spending time in Vietnam and witnessing tragic deaths as a result of plague, his interest in the science of *Yersinia pestis* grew, and he began years of research on this and many other diseases. He became one of the most prominent plague researchers in the world.

During a 2001 trip to Tanzania, Butler collected numerous quantities of sample plague from patients who had contracted the disease and proceeded to bring the samples back into the United States, claiming he was unaware of CDC policy on pathogen transport. In January 2002, Butler filed a report to his university claiming 30 of 150 vials of plague were missing from his lab. The university, concerned about a possible terrorist-backed theft, called the FBI. With no signs of forced entry or foul play, investigators began to question Butler and his involvement in the case. After 2 days of interrogation, Butler admitted to destroying the vials himself and was then taken to a Lubbock jail and charged with lying to federal agents about the disappearance of the vials and illegally bringing samples of plague into the United States.

Thomas Butler, denying a plea bargain, was charged with 18 counts of theft, fraud, and embezzlement; 13 counts of mail fraud; 13 counts of wire fraud; and 3 counts of unauthorized export. He was convicted and sentenced to 2 years in prison and more than $50,000 in fines. He was stripped of his medical license, and, despite pleas from prominent scientists around the world, he served his time in jail and his career was destroyed.

Whether the FBI was making an example out of Dr. Butler, whether foul play was involved, or whether the cavalier ways of disease researchers had to be amended in the post-9/11 world, this case was a wake-up call to researchers around the country. This case shook researchers into understanding that their roles and responsibilities as scientists have changed, and the consequences of nonadherence to the rules is significant.

Sources: Chang K. 30 Plague vials put career on line. *New York Times.* October 19, 2003. Available at: http://www.nytimes.com/2003/10/19/us/30-plague-vials-put-career-on-line.html. Accessed October 9, 2010; Enserink M, Malakoff D. The trials of Thomas Butler. *Science.* December 2003;302(5653):2054–2063; and Chang K. Scientist in plague case is sentenced to two years. *New York Times.* March 11, 2004. Available at: http://www.nytimes.com/2004/03/11/us/scientist-in-plague-case-is-sentenced-to-two-years.html. Accessed October 9, 2010.

---

and systems that do not naturally exist.[29] What this means is that biologists and engineers, along with computer modelers and other experts, combine expertise to synthesize biological agents. These efforts can be rapid, relatively inexpensive, and efficient for the creation of drugs and other medical countermeasures. The process also, however, can be used to synthesize naturally occurring pathogens de novo, including pathogens that are difficult to obtain or have been eradicated. It is also possible to use this process to create novel biological agents with unique properties.

The U.S. government sees synthetic biology as an important scientific development with potential applications for the advancement of health and technology. There is also recognition that the potential for misuse exists. The NSABB has released reports addressing the biosecurity concerns raised by synthetic biology,[30] the National Academies of Science has reviewed the topic,[31] and the scientific and policy community continues to work on how best to address the dual-use implications for synthetic biology.

COOPERATIVE THREAT REDUCTION

One of the ways the government has sought to reduce the biological threat has been to engage in what are called *cooperative threat reduction* (CTR) programs. These programs started out as an effort to contain the proliferation of former Soviet biological weapons expertise. The idea was for scientists in the former weapons facilities to be redirected from working on biological weapons to using their skills to improve life sciences and health, to dismantle the former offensive weapons facilities, and to rebuild facilities to advance science and help the local population, like vaccine manufacturing plants.

These programs continued throughout the former Soviet Union (FSU) for years. They also eventually moved into pathogen security and creating laboratory infrastructure to contain agents and reduce the potential for theft. In the 2000s, the program began to move out of the FSU and into other parts of the world with identified threats. The programs were expanded to places such as Pakistan and Indonesia, which had laboratories, scientists, and agents (not well secured) and where significant security threat existed, particularly from terrorist organizations.

In the past few years, these CTR programs have expanded to address other aspects related to containing biological threats, including—significantly—the strengthening of disease surveillance capacity through laboratory construction, workforce development, and systems strengthening, and the program has moved to regions where the burden of disease is great and the infrastructure for surveillance and response is weak, including areas of sub-Saharan Africa. While many government organizations are involved in these efforts, the primary funders for the program are the DoD, through the Defense Threat Reduction Agency (DTRA), and the Department of State's Biological Engagement Program (BEP).

KEY WORDS

Biosecurity
Biosafety
Biorisk management
Dual-use dilemma
National Science Advisory Board for Biosecurity
Select agents
Synthetic biology
Cooperative threat reduction

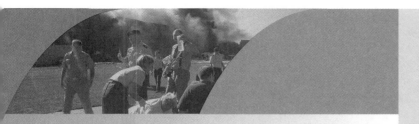

Discussion Questions

1. What is the difference among biosecurity, biosafety, and biorisk management?

2. Explain the dual-use dilemma.

3. Who should be responsible for policing the publication of scientific papers for potential dual use? Should there be any policing?

4. Would you have published the papers that were reviewed by NSABB? Why or why not?

5. How should scientists and policy makers best manage advances in life sciences against the possible misuse of science?

6. Do you think CTR programs are effective? If so, should they be expanded?

REFERENCES

1. Salerno RM, Koelm JG. *Biological Laboratory and Transporation Security and the Biological Weapons Convention*. Sandia National Laboratories. February 2002. Available at: http://www.cmc.sandia.gov/cmc-papers/sand2002-1067p.pdf. Accessed September 19, 2010.

2. Committee on Laboratory Security and Personnel Reliability Assurance Systems for Laboratories Conducting Research on Biological Select Agents and Toxins, National Research Council of the National Academies. Introduction: The promise and performance of BSAT research. *Responsible Research with Biological Select Agents and Toxins*. Washington, DC: The National Academies Press; 2009. Available at: http://books.nap.edu/openbook.php?record_id=12774&page=27.

3. World Health Organization. *Biorisk Management: Laboratory Biosecurity Guidance*. September 2006. Available at: http://www.who.int/csr/resources/publications/biosafety/WHO_CDS_EPR_2006_6.pdf. Accessed September 19, 2010.

4. Committee on Education on Dual Use Issues in the Life Sciences, National Research Council of the National Academies. Introduction: The life sciences and dual use issues. *Challenges and Opportunities for Education about Dual Use Issues in the Life Sciences*. Washington, DC : The National Academies Press; 2010.

5. National Institutes of Health, Office of Biotechnology Activities. Dual use research and dual use research of concern. *Dual Use Research and the National Science Advisory Board for Biosecurity: Frequently Asked Questions*. Available at: http://oba.od.nih.gov/oba/faqs/NSABB%20FAQs%20NEW%20FINAL71910.pdf. Accessed September 19, 2010.

6. President's Scientific Research Board; John R. Steelman, Chair. *Science and Public Policy: A Program for the Nation*. August 27, 1947.

7. Kerr, Larry, National Institutes of Health. Integrating science and security: Making intelligent decisions. *National Institutes of Health Webcast*. September 28, 2006. Available at: http://videocast.nih.gov/Summary.asp?File=13387. Accessed September 20, 2010.

8. President Harry S. Truman. President Harry S. Truman's address to the Centennial Anniversary AAAS Meeting (1948). National Science Foundation. September 1948. Available at: http://www.nsf.gov/about/history/nsf50/truman1948_address.jsp. Accessed September 19, 2010.

9. Committee on a New Government—University Partnership for Science and Security Committee on Science, Technology, and Law, National Research Council of the National Academies. Policies for openness and information control. *Science and Security in a Post 9/11 World: A Report Based on Regional Discussions Between the Science and Security Communities*. Washington, DC: The National Academies Press; 2007.

10. Schweitzer G. Who wins in U.S.–Soviet science ventures? *Bulletin of the Atomic Scientists*. October 1988;5(8):28–32.

11. Federation of American Scientists. Executive Order 12356—National Security Information. April 2, 1982. Available at: http://www.fas.org/irp/offdocs/eo12356.htm. Accessed September 19, 2010.

12. Panel on Scientific Communication and National Security, Committee on Science, Engineering, and Public Policy, National Academy of Sciences, National Academy of Engineering, Institute of Medicine. *Scientific Communication and National Security*. Washington, DC: National Academy Press; 1982.

13. Federation of American Scientists. NSDD-189: *National Policy on the Transfer of Scientific, Technical and Engineering Information*. September 21, 1985. Available at: http://www.fas.org/irp/offdocs/nsdd/nsdd-189.htm. Accessed September 19, 2010.

14. Marburger, Dr. John H., Director of the Office of Science and Technology Policy, Executive Office of the White House. *Conducting Research During the War on Terrorism: Balancing Openness and Security*. Written testimony in hearing before the House of Representatives Committee on Science; October 10, 2002; 107th Congress, Second Session.

15. Rice C. Letter from National Security Advisor to CSIS. Council on Governmental Relations. November 1, 2001. Available at: www.cogr.edu/viewDoc.cfm?DocID=151621. Accessed September 19, 2010.

16. Jackson RJ, Ramsay AJ, Christensen CD, Beaton S, Hall DF, Ramshaw IA. Expression of mouse interleukin-4 by a recombinant ectromelia virus suppresses cytolytic lymphocyte responses and overcomes genetic resistance to mousepox. *Journal of Virology*. February 2001;75(3):1205–1210.

17. Selgelid MJ, Weir L. The mousepox experience: An interview with Ronald Jackson and Ian Ramshaw on dual-use research. *EMBO reports*. January 2010;11(1):18–24.

18. Cello J, Paul AV, Wimmer E. Chemical synthesis of poliovirus cDNA: Generation of infectious virus in the absence of natural template. *Science*. August 2002;297(5583):1016–1018.

19. Parkhill J, Wren BW, Thomson NR, et al. Genome sequence of Yersinia pestis, the causative agent of plague. *Nature*. October 2001; 413(6855):523–527.

20. Shea DA. CRS report for Congress: Balancing scientific publication and national security concerns: Issues for Congress. *Federation of American Scientists*. July 9, 2003. Available at: http://www.fas.org/irp/crs/RL31695.pdf. Accessed September 19, 2010.

21. Sharp PA. 1918 flu and responsible science. *Science*. October 2005;310(5745):17.

22. Kurzweil R, Joy B. Recipe for destruction. *New York Times*. October 17, 2005. Available at: http://www.nytimes.com/2005/10/17/opinion/17kurzweiljoy.html. Accessed September 19, 2010.

23. Wein LM, Liu Y. Analyzing a bioterror attack on the food supply: The case of botulinum toxin in milk. *PNAS*. July 2005;102(28):9984–9989.

24. Steneck NH. *Introduction to the Responsible Conduct of Research*. U.S. Department of Health and Human Services, Office of Research Integrity. August 2007. Available at: http://ori.dhhs.gov/documents/rcrintro.pdf. Accessed September 19, 2010.

25. Antiterrorism and Effective Death Penalty Act of 1996; Public Law No. 104-132.

26. Committee on Science, Engineering, and Public Policy, National Academy of Sciences, National Academy of Engineering, Institute of Medicine. *On Being a Scientist: Responsible Conduct in Research*. Washington, DC: National Academy Press; 1995.

27. Uniting and Strengthening America by Providing Appropriate Tools Required to Intercept and Obstruct Terrorism (USA PATRIOT) Act of 2001; Public Law No. 107-56.

28. The White House, Office of the Press Secretary. Executive Order—Optimizing the Security of Biological Select Agents and Toxins in the United States. July 2, 2010. Available at: http://www.whitehouse.gov/the-press-office/executive-order-optimizing-security-biological-select-agents-and-toxins-united-stat. Accessed September 19, 2010.

29. Synthetic Biology community. *Synthetic Biology*. Available at: http://syntheticbiology.org/. Accessed September 19, 2010.

30. National Science Advisory Board for Biosecurity (NSABB). *Addressing Biosecurity Concerns Related to Synthetic Biology*. April 2010. Available at: http://oba.od.nih.gov/biosecurity/pdf/NSABB%20SynBio%20DRAFT%20Report-FINAL%20(2)_6-7-10.pdf. Accessed December 2, 2010.

31. The National Academies' Committee on Science, Technology, and Law. Opportunities and challenges in the emerging field of synthetic biology: A symposium. *The National Academies' Committee on Science, Technology, and Law, Policy and Global Affairs*. July 9–10, 2009. Available at: http://sites.nationalacademies.org/pga/stl/PGA_050738. Accessed December 2, 2010.

CHAPTER **8**

The Research Agenda

INTRODUCTION

Thus far, we have been examining the overall effort to defend against, prepare for, and respond to public health emergencies. In this chapter, we turn our attention to the research community. From basic scientific research to the development of medical countermeasures, the scientific and pharmaceutical communities are integral components of public health preparedness. We will look at each of the federal agencies engaged in supporting the preparedness research agenda. This chapter will examine the infrastructure associated with supporting basic scientific research related to public health preparedness, including the types of laboratories necessary and the responsibilities of researchers. We will also explore the public health emergency medical countermeasures enterprise (PHEMCE) and related activities to document the policies and challenges associated with research, development, and distribution of

drugs and vaccines that may be necessary in response to an emergency or public health disaster.

BASIC SCIENTIFIC RESEARCH

Most of the basic scientific research in support of public health preparedness, and addressing the CBRN threat, is led through funding of grants and contracts by the National Institutes of Health (NIH), specifically, the National Institute of Allergy and Infectious Diseases (NIAID). NIH, through its intramural research program and extramural grants, supports the advancement of scientific knowledge that can lead to future treatments (therapeutics and vaccines) and diagnostics. Research that might not obviously be linked to potential threats can often prove valuable. For example, NIH funded research into coronaviruses for years. When SARS emerged in 2003, and a coronavirus was identified as the causative agent, scientific expertise regarding this relatively obscure virus was ready and available because of long-term funding by the NIH. NIAID supports research into the basic biology and pathogenesis of threat agents, many of which are not well understood. In addition, NIAID supports research on host response to threat agents and toxins, immunity, and cross-disciplinary research that can lead to vaccines, therapies, and diagnostics (see **Figure 8-1**).[1] The focus of this research is less of a "one bug–one drug" approach and instead aims to use a more flexible, broad-spectrum approach that enables development of medical countermeasures that might be effective against a variety of agents, technology that could be applied to whole classes of products, and platforms that might reduce the time and expenses associated with creating products.[2] **Box 8-1** lists the multitude of research strategies and reports produced by NIH in support of preparedness and WMD defense.

In addition to federal support for basic research on biological organisms and toxins, NIAID also supports research that leads to medical countermeasures for exposure to ionizing radiation and works with the National Institute of Neurological Disorders and Stroke (NINDS), the National Institute of Environmental Health Sciences (NIEHS), and other parts of NIH to support efforts that lead to the development of medical countermeasures for exposure to chemical threats.[3]

INFRASTRUCTURE FOR RESEARCH

Over the past 10 years, to support the growing research agenda to address CBRN and naturally occurring threats, as well as

BOX 8-1 NIH and NIAID Research Strategies and Expert Reports for Biodefense, Chemical Defense, and Radiological Defense

Biodefense
- NIAID Strategic Plan for Biodefense Research
- NIAID Biodefense Research Agenda for CDC Category A Agents
- NIAID Biodefense Research Agenda for Category B and C Priority Pathogens

Chemical and Toxin Defense
- NIH Strategic Plan and Research Agenda for Medical Countermeasures against Chemical Threats
- NIAID Expert Panel Review on Medical Chemical Defense
- NIAID Expert Panel on Botulinum Toxins
- NIAID Expert Panel on Botulinum Diagnostics
- NIAID Expert Panel on Botulinum Neurotoxins Therapeutics

Radiological and Nuclear Defense
- NIH Strategic Plan and Research Agenda for Medical Countermeasures against Radiological and Nuclear Threats, June 2005

Source: All reports available on the NIAID website. U.S. Department of Health and Human Services. National Institute of Allergy and Infectious Diseases. *Biodefense & Related Programs.* November 16, 2009. Available at: http://www.niaid.nih.gov/topics/biodefenserelated/pages/default.aspx. Accessed August 23, 2010.

FIGURE 8-1 Biodefense Research: NIAID Approach to How Basic Scientific Research Leads to Vaccines, Therapies, and Diagnostics

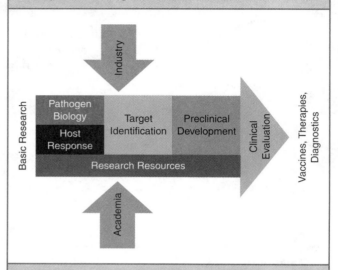

Source: Reproduced from the National Institute of Allergy and Infectious Disease. Biodefense: Introduction to Biodefense Research. Available at: http://www.niaid.nih.gov/topics/BiodefenseRelated/Biodefense/research/Pages/Introduction.aspx

to develop domestic diagnostic capacity, the U.S. government has invested in building laboratory infrastructure, including high-containment research laboratories, such as BSL 3s and 4s. (See Chapter 7, Table 7-1 for a description of BSL laboratory distinctions, and **Figure 8-2** for what it looks like to work inside such a facility.)

Both DHHS (mostly through NIH) and DHS have supported the expansion of the research infrastructure through support for BSL 3s and BSL 4s, as well as Centers of Excellence around the country. There are currently 13 BSL 4 facilities in the United States; 11 if the Galveston labs are counted together and the facility at the NIH main campus is excluded:

- Centers for Disease Control and Prevention in Atlanta, Georgia (DHHS/CDC facility).
- Robert E. Shope, MD Laboratory, Galveston, Texas (university facility).
- Galveston National Laboratory, Galveston, Texas (DHHS/NIAID facility at University of Texas Medical Branch). (Note: The Shope Laboratory and the Galveston National Laboratory are run contiguously and may not always be counted as separate entities.)
- U.S. Army Medical Research Institute for Infectious Diseases, Frederick, Maryland (DoD facility).

FIGURE 8-2 Laboratorians Working in a BSL 4 Facility

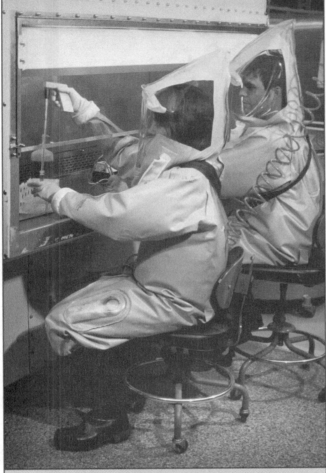

Source: Reproduced from CDC Public Health Image Library; CDC/ Jim Gathany.

- Southwest Foundation for Biomedical Research, San Antonio, Texas (private facility).
- Rocky Mountain Laboratories Integrated Research Facility, Hamilton, Montana (DHHS/NIAID facility).
- Georgia State University, Atlanta, Georgia (university facility, not a full BSL 4 facility; glove box capability).
- National Biodefense Analysis and Countermeasures Center, Frederick, Maryland (DHS facility). Note: This is not yet operational; it is a planned facility.
- Integrated Research Facility, Frederick, Maryland (DHHS/NIAID facility). Note: This is not yet operational; it is a planned facility.

- Virginia Division of Consolidated Laboratory Services, Richmond, Virginia [Virginia Department of Health Facility (BSL 4 surge capacity)].
- National Bio and Agro-Defense Facility, Manhattan, Kansas (DHS facility). Note: This is not yet operational; it is a planned facility.
- National Biocontainment Laboratory, Boston, Massachusetts (DHHS/NIAID facility at Boston University). Note: This is not yet operational; it is a planned facility.
- National Institutes of Health, Bethesda, Maryland (DHHS/NIAID). Note: This is a small BSL 4 facility on the NIH main campus. This facility, however, is only operated at a BSL 3 level.

Much of the federal biodefense work is centralized at Fort Detrick in Frederick, Maryland. (See **Figure 8-3**.) DHS centralizes its research at the National Biodefense Analysis and Countermeasures Center (NBACC) located on the Fort Detrick campus. The official mission of NBACC is to "provide the nation with the scientific basis for characterization of biological threats and bioforensic analysis to support attribution of their use against the American public."[4] This center focuses on activities that support threat characterization, as well as bioforensic analysis to support attribution assessments of biocrimes and bioterrorism.[4] Also at Fort Detrick is the U.S. Army Medical Research Institute for Infectious Diseases (USAMRIID), a BSL 4 facility that has long engaged in biodefense work and basic scientific research, including research on dangerous pathogens, such as Ebola. USDA and the NIH/National Cancer Institute (NCI) have also long had a presence on the campus. Recently, NIAID constructed an integrated research facility (IRF) to direct, coordinate, and facilitate research in emerging infectious diseases and biodefense to support countermeasure development and improve medical outcomes.[5]

DHHS and DHS both have a network of centers around the country that engage in and support research. These Centers of Excellence focus on countering threats to national security, including those posed by emerging infectious diseases and CBRN agents. NIH supports Regional Centers of Excellence (RCEs) for biodefense and emerging infectious diseases. (See **Figure 8-4**.) These centers provide infrastructures for BSL 3 laboratories and animal studies, provide training, and engage in basic research in preclinical activities, immunological techniques, and aerobiology.[6] There are currently 11 centers around the country. In addition, NIH also supports 13 Regional Biocontainment Laboratories at the BSL 2/3 level, which form a key part of the national response network.

FIGURE 8-3 National Interagency Confederation for Biological Research

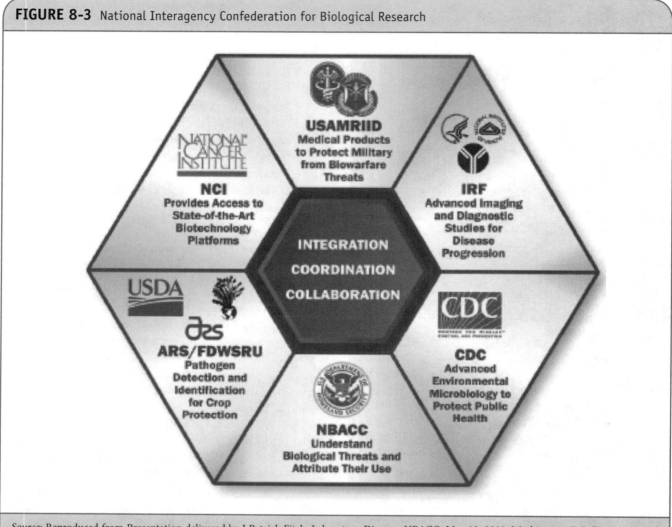

Source: Reproduced from Presentation delivered by J Patrick Fitch, Laboratory Director NBACC. May 12, 2008, Washington, DC. "Science-Based Biodefense Analysis in an Uncertain World" http://csis.org/files/media/csis/events/080529_csis_fitch_presentation.pdf

DHS also supports a network of primarily university-based Centers of Excellence (COE), funded by the Science and Technology Directorate, Office of Research and Development. They are listed in **Box 8-2**. Each COE has specific goals and objectives, including technology improvements, basic research, and multidisciplinary analysis.

HIGH-CONTAINMENT LABORATORIES—THE DEBATE

Earlier we discussed the expansion of laboratory infrastructure in the past decade. While the government has invested in this infrastructure—citing a need for more laboratory resources, enhanced research, and diagnostic facilities—others have pointed to a "proliferation of laboratories" and brought

up security and environmental concerns associated with having so many high containment laboratories. Questions arose as to:

- How much laboratory capacity is sufficient?
- Is or was there enough coordination among federal funding agencies in determining where these labs should be built?
- Does increasing the number of labs increase the potential for intentional or accidental spread of dangerous pathogens?[7]

On September 22, 2009, the U.S. House of Representatives Subcommittee on Oversight and Investigations, Committee on Energy and Commerce, held a hearing on federal oversight

FIGURE 8-4 Map of the 11 NIH-Supported Regional Centers of Excellence

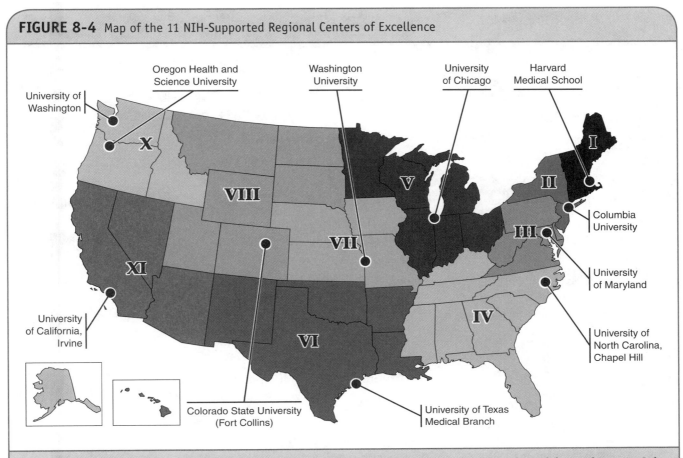

University of
Washington

Oregon Health and
Science University

Washington
University

University
of Chicago

Harvard
Medical School

Columbia
University

University
of Maryland

University
of California,
Irvine

University of
North Carolina,
Chapel Hill

Colorado State University
(Fort Collins)

University of Texas
Medical Branch

Source: Reproduced from the National Institute of Allergy and Infectious Disease. Regional Centers of Excellence for Biodefense and Emerging Infectious Diseases. Available at: http://www.niaid.nih.gov/labsandresources/resources/rce/pages/sites.aspx

of high-containment biolaboratories. This was a follow-up hearing to one held two years earlier, on October 4, 2007, and the main question at both of those hearings was How many high containment labs are there in the United States?[8] While we know how many laboratories work with select agents and are registered with either the CDC or the USDA (286 total),[7] there is still no answer to the question of how many total laboratories there are with BSL 3 capabilities. This is partially because many different entities oversee BSL 3 laboratories and no single agency is in charge of keeping track of just how many exist, which brings up additional questions of how they can be regulated.

Galveston and Boston

In 2002, NIAID hosted several blue ribbon panels of experts, who recommended expanding the research infrastructure to include the construction and renovation of BSL 3 and BSL 4

laboratories. NIAID decided to fund the construction of two National Biocontainment Laboratories, capable of doing BSL 4 research. In fiscal year 2003, Boston University and the University of Texas Medical Branch (UTMB) at Galveston were chosen in a national competitive process to be the sites for the two BSL 4 laboratories.[9]

What followed is an interesting case study in public relations, community engagement, and political support. Galveston, a location prone to hurricanes, made a strong argument about how hurricanes were predictable, a facility could be built to withstand them, and Galveston was—in fact—an ideal site for a facility. UTMB worked closely with the community, developed support for the project from the bottom up, and, as of 2010, has a fully functional facility that has already proven its ability to withstand hurricanes.

In Boston, university officials obtained support from high-level political officials for the location of the BSL 4

BOX 8-2   DHS Centers of Excellence

1. The Center for Risk and Economic Analysis of Terrorism Events (CREATE), led by the University of Southern California

2. The Center for Advancing Microbial Risk Assessment (CAMRA), led by Michigan State University and Drexel University

3. The National Center for Foreign Animal and Zoonotic Disease Defense (FAZD), led by Texas A&M University

4. The National Center for Food Protection and Defense (NCFPD), led by the University of Minnesota

5. The National Consortium for the Study of Terrorism and Responses to Terrorism (START), led by the University of Maryland

6. The National Center for the Study of Preparedness and Catastrophic Event Response (PACER), led by Johns Hopkins University

7. The Center of Excellence for Awareness & Location of Explosives-Related Threats (ALERT), led by Northeastern University and the University of Rhode Island

8. The National Center for Border Security and Immigration, led by the University of Arizona in Tucson (research co-lead) and the University of Texas at El Paso (education co-lead)

9. The Center for Maritime, Island and Port Security, led by the University of Hawaii and Stevens Institute of Technology

10. The Center for Natural Disasters, Coastal Infrastructure, and Emergency Management, led by the University of North Carolina at Chapel Hill and Jackson State University

11. The National Transportation Security Center of Excellence (NTSCOE). It comprises seven institutions:
    - Connecticut Transportation Institute at the University of Connecticut
    - Tougaloo College
    - Texas Southern University
    - National Transit Institute at Rutgers—The State University of New Jersey
    - Homeland Security Management Institute at Long Island University
    - Mack Blackwell National Rural Transportation Study Center at the University of Arkansas
    - Mineta Transportation Institute at San José State University

12. The Center of Excellence in Command, Control and Interoperability (C2I), led by Purdue University (visualization sciences co-lead) and Rutgers University (data sciences co-lead)

Source: U.S. Department of Homeland Security. *Homeland Security Centers of Excellence.* November 12, 2009. Available at: http://www.dhs.gov/files/programs/editorial_0498.shtm. Accessed October 9, 2010.

facility but made only minimal effort to engage the community. Limited attention was paid to environmental assessments or to working with the local neighborhoods to educate them about the risks associated with having a BSL 4 facility in the middle of an urban community. The community reacted very negatively, and construction on the facility was blocked by court order. As of fall 2010, the facility has been constructed, but it will not be allowed to become operational as a BSL 4 until a third risk assessment is complete and the courts approve operations.

Increasing high-containment laboratory capacity has been described as a double-edged sword.[7] Building capacity allows for more research, more infrastructure for diagnostic testing, and advancement of scientific knowledge in general. On the other hand, increasing the number of labs means increasing the number of personnel working in these labs—which increases the opportunities for accidental exposures to pathogens, mistakes, or accidents that might lead to environmental release of pathogens; or for a research scientist to intentionally access a pathogen and use it for malevolent purposes; or for personnel to share knowledge with an outside entity or person who then uses that knowledge for malevolent purposes.

These high-containment laboratories are heavily regulated in the United States. There are physical security measures, as well as personal responsibilities, all aimed at limiting both accidents and potential intentional-use events. One question still debated, though, is the level of oversight required of laboratory personnel. Currently, personnel who work with select agents are required to have a background check. There is no such requirement for personnel who do not work with select agents.

MEDICAL COUNTERMEASURES

One of the primary objectives listed in the 2009 National Health Security Strategy (see Chapter 3) was the need to promote a process to develop, buy, and distribute medical countermeasures.[10] The policies, strategies, and methodologies behind the development and delivery of medical countermeasures have developed over the decade and are now part of what is known as the Public Health Emergency Medical Countermeasures Enterprise (PHEMCE).

As we saw in Chapter 6, the Project Bioshield Act was passed in 2004, with the purpose of establishing a market to purchase medical countermeasures to treat exposures to biological, chemical, or radiological agents. A special reserve fund was established, with $5.6 billion to be used over 10 years, to purchase these countermeasures to put into the Strategic National Stockpile.[11] The federal government, usually through NIH, was able to provide funding for the initial research associated with discovery and valuation. Drug development companies were then on their own to move the initial discovery into a tested, safe product—a process that might take up to 10 years—before the government could provide funds again to do final testing and purchase the product. In addition, the act did not provide companies with liability protection if a product was used for emergency purposes but had not yet completed all final stages of approval by the FDA. (This problem was addressed by passage of the PREP Act in 2005; see Chapter 6.) As a result, few companies were willing to invest in the development of products.

The 2006 PAHPA legislation addressed some of the problems in the Project Bioshield Act, allowing companies to receive payments before delivery of the product, which enables them to move a product through testing with financial support. PAHPA also established the Biomedical Advanced Research and Development Authority (BARDA), which sits in DHHS/ASPR to manage the development of medical countermeasures against CBRN threats, emerging infections, and pandemic influenza.[12(Title IV)] At about the same time, DHHS established PHEMCE (see **Box 8-3**) to coordinate the planning and execution of developing medical countermeasures across organizations.

The federal process for PHEMCE starts with DHS, which is tasked with conducting risk and threat assessments and creating a list of agents and conditions. These agents and conditions then become the priorities for the development of medical countermeasures, and DHHS directs that countermeasures be produced to counter these threats.

NIH and NIAID in particular then fund basic and applied research to address the threat list. When basic science leads to the potential for a medical countermeasure, BARDA becomes involved to manage advanced product development. Throughout the drug development process, FDA provides review and regulatory oversight and eventual approval for licensing. Products are acquired through Project Bioshield, which are then transferred to CDC, where the countermeasures are stored and maintained. CDC continues to manage

---

BOX 8-3 Public Health Emergency Medical Countermeasures Strategy

1. Enhance regulatory innovation, science, and capacity.

2. Improve domestic manufacturing capacity.

3. Provide advanced development and manufacturing services to development partners.

4. Create new ways for the enterprise to work with partners.

5. Develop financial incentives.

6. Address roadblocks, from concept to advanced development.

7. Improve management and administration.

Source: U.S. Department of Health and Human Services, Assistant Secretary for Preparedness and Response. *The Public Health Emergency Medical Countermeasures Enterprise Review, Transforming the Enterprise to Meet Long-Range National Needs.* August 2010. Available at: http://www.hhs.gov/nvpo/nvac/meetings/upcomingmeetings/korch_presentation.pdf. Accessed December 10, 2010.

acquisition after the product becomes part of the Strategic National Stockpile (SNS). If the agent then has to be utilized, CDC is in charge of releasing it from the SNS, and DHHS is in charge of coordinating deployment and utilization.[2,13]

Stockpiling and Distribution of Medical Countermeasures

In 1999, CDC established what was known as the National Pharmaceutical Stockpile (NPS); it was renamed the Strategic National Stockpile in 2003. The purpose of the SNS is to amass and store large amounts of drugs, vaccines, and medical equipment that can rapidly be deployed to any locality in the country in response to a public health emergency. Once federal officials determine that an emergency exists and that SNS assets should be deployed, an initial delivery of drugs, antidotes, and supplies can be made to any state in the country within 12 hours. An additional shipment, if necessary, can be available in 24 to 36 hours. CDC, in collaboration with the rest of the PHEMCE partners, determines what should be in the stockpile and ensures the material has not expired.[14]

Cities Readiness Initiative

When the SNS is deployed, it is the responsibility of state and local officials to accept the material, store it, and distribute it to the affected population. The Cities Readiness Initiative (CRI) is a federally funded program to help prepare local entities to respond to a public health emergency and develop distribution plans for getting needed medical supplies and countermeasures to their populations. The CRI program was established in 2004 and now funds 72 metropolitan statistical areas. CDC provides technical assistance to the 72 sites so that they can effectively and efficiently receive items from the SNS, store them, and deliver them.

MedKit

One drug distribution method currently being evaluated is called MedKit. This is a prepackaged kit of medication—5-day supply of antibiotics—that would be delivered to individual households for safekeeping. Then, if an event occurred, the population would be directed to take the medication. Initial studies have indicated significant cooperation on the part of the public to treat the medication responsibly, and federal agencies, including the FDA, continue to evaluate this as a preparedness option.[15]

U.S. Postal Service

Possibly one of the most interesting preparedness tactics is to use the U.S. Postal Service (USPS) to assist in the distribution of medical countermeasures. If an event happens, it may be imperative to get medical countermeasures to the population within 24 to 72 hours to prevent large-scale morbidity and mortality. By an Executive Order on December 30, 2009, President Obama ordered DHHS and DHS to work with USPS to establish a national USPS medical countermeasures dispensing model.[16] Recognizing that an emergency requiring the USPS to distribute medical countermeasures may likely be an event that inspires fear and panic in the population, the EO also calls for a plan to have law enforcement officials escorting postal service employees to secure the countermeasures and provide for the safety of the delivery men and women.

ONGOING RESEARCH DEBATES

As the federal government continues to support the research and development of medical countermeasures, the research community struggles with a series of challenges associated with preparedness and biodefense research. Some question the necessity of classifying any research findings. Some academics continue to voice concern over the severity of some of the regulations placed on them for security concerns, while others argue that there are not enough regulations to ensure research is conducted safely and securely. One of the most interesting and hotly debated issues has been whether to destroy the remaining stockpiles of smallpox. (See **Box 8-4**.)

At the end of this chapter, we include a reprint of an illustrated guide produced by Galveston National Laboratory on what a scientist must do to work in a BSL 4 laboratory (see **Figure 8-5**). Obviously, the purpose of this book is not to prepare readers to work in a BSL 4 laboratory, but we thought readers might be interested in what is involved in working in one of these facilities to better understand the safety and security measures taken, as well as the responsibilities of researchers working with very dangerous pathogens.

KEY WORDS

Public Health Emergency Medical Countermeasures Enterprise
Biomedical research
High-containment laboratories
Fort Detrick
National Biodefense Analysis and Countermeasures Center
Centers of Excellence
Medical countermeasures
Strategic National Stockpile
Cities Readiness Initiative
MedKit

BOX 8-4 Smallpox Destruction Debate

In 1966, the World Health Organization (WHO) launched an international campaign to eradicate smallpox. After 11 years, they succeeded, making it one of the most profound public health accomplishments to date. Following eradication, there was a laboratory accident in 1978 that led to two infections and one fatality. This lab incident led the World Health Assembly to pass Resolution 33.4 in 1980, which urged all countries to destroy their smallpox stocks or transfer them to one of the four designated collaborating centers established by WHO.* Three years following Resolution 33.4, CDC in Atlanta and the State Research Institute for Viral Preparations in Moscow (Vector) were named the exclusive repositories of the smallpox virus.

Despite naming Vector and CDC as the only two repositories of smallpox in the world, evidence was compiled that the virus was not only in multiple countries—including Iran, Iraq, and North Korea—but that it was potentially being used to develop biological weapons.** In addition, inspectors found evidence that the Soviet Union had transferred the smallpox to an offensive biological weapons facility and was using it as part of their offensive biological weapons program. Following the collapse of the Soviet Union, security experts worried that smallpox samples may have left the country. By 1996, the concern about undetected stocks had increased, and Resolution 49.10 was adopted by the WHO, recommending that all smallpox virus stocks be destroyed by June 30, 1999. However, concerns of a possible bioterrorist attack and the need for more antiviral drugs and vaccines in preparation for such an event led the CDC to reconsider the resolution and to conserve the remaining stocks.

With influence and scientific backing from the Institute of Medicine, the WHO established a three-year program (Resolution 52.10) that allowed for applied research with the smallpox virus at the two authorized repositories, for the benefit of public health. At the end of the three-year research period in 2002, the WHO passed Resolution 55.15, which extended the smallpox research for an indefinite period of time until all research goals and needs have been accomplished.

By 2006, most of the research goals had been fulfilled, and, as a result, 46 member-states of the WHO drafted a resolution to have the final smallpox stocks in Vector and the CDC destroyed by June 30, 2010. However, the United States, Russia, and multiple other countries blocked the resolution. This led to Resolution 60.1 the following year, which claimed the need for a consensus on the issue of the smallpox destruction and helped with the recent decision to have a major review in 2010. This review gave guidance to the World Health Assembly (WHA) of May 2011, where a final conclusion was planned to be made on the destruction of the smallpox stocks.

Retentionists (those in favor of preserving the last two remaining smallpox stocks) claim that the potential for a smallpox outbreak comes more from the threat of unknown stocks or from de novo synthesis and not from the two remaining repositories holding the smallpox virus. They also argue that research is still needed to create novel ways to contain the virus in the event there is a bioterrorist attack leading to a smallpox pandemic.

In contrast to the retentionists, those opposed to the saving of the smallpox virus, known as destructionists, believe that an accidental outbreak could cause devastation, leaving the most efficient prevention of this type of incident to be the destruction of the virus. Further, they strongly believe in the "insider threat," represented as a scientist with access to the smallpox virus at either of the repositories using that access to bring the virus to outside, dangerous sources.

Delegates at the 2011 WHA meeting agreed to retain stockpiles for now, and review this debate again in several years.

---

* The global distribution of laboratories reporting possession of the smallpox virus to the WHO in 1975 was as follows: Africa (5), Americas (18), Southeast Asia (13), Europe (29), eastern Mediterranean (3), and western Pacific (6). Although China did not respond to the WHO survey, samples of the smallpox virus were then held at the Institute for the Control of Drugs and Biological Products in Beijing, bringing the total number of laboratory stocks to 75.

** In the aftermath of the 2003 Iraq War, the U.S.-led Iraq Survey Group failed to find conclusive evidence that Iraq had possessed stocks of the smallpox virus.

Sources: Fenner F, Hendemon DA, Arita I, Jezek Z, Ladnyi ID. *Smallpox and Its Eradication.* Geneva: World Health Organization, 1988; Gellman B. 4 Nations Thought to Possess Smallpox: Iraq, N. Korea Named, Two Officials Say. *The Washington Post.* November 5, 2002. Available at: http://www.washingtonpost.com/wp-dyn/content/article/2006/06/12/AR2006061200704.html. Accessed October 9, 2010; Mangold T, Goldberg J. *Plague Wars: The Terrifying Reality of Biological Warfare.* New York: St. Martin's Press, 1999; Committee on the Assessment of Future Scientific Needs for Live Variola Virus, Board on Global Health, Institute of Medicine. *Assessment of Future Scientific Needs for Live Variola Virus.* Washington, DC: National Academies Press, 1999; World Health Organization. Smallpox Eradication: Destruction of Variola Virus Stocks, WHA60.1, Agenda Item 12.2, Sixtieth World Health Assembly. May 18, 2007. Available at: http://apps.who.int/gb/ebwha/pdf_files/WHA60/A60_R1-en.pdf. Accessed October 9, 2010; and U.S. Department of State. *Adherence to and Compliance with Arms Control, Nonproliferation, and Disarmament Agreements and Commitments.* July 2010. Available at: http://www.state.gov/documents/organization/145181.pdf. Accessed October 9, 2010.

FIGURE 8-5 What a Scientist Must Do to Work in a BSL 4 Laboratory

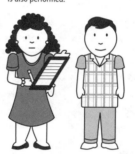

Getting approval:

1 Four to six months prior to requested access to select agents [see "Terms"], the FBI will do extensive background checks on the scientist.

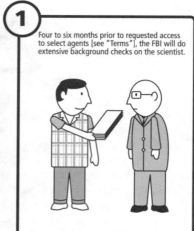

2 The scientist undergoes an initial health assessment.

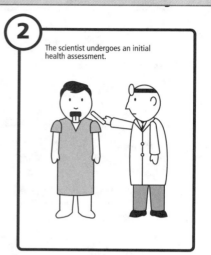

3 The scientist is evaluated for laboratory experience (BSL2 experience required), as well as biosafety experience and knowledge. A laboratory skills assessment is also performed.

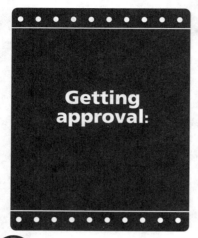

4 The scientist must complete preliminary biosafety training.

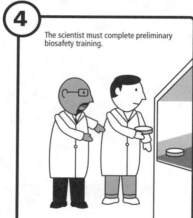

5 A supervised BSL3 training period of one to six months is required, followed by three to six months of solo BSL3 work experience, depending upon previous BSL3 experience.

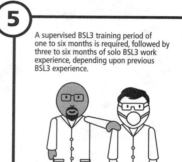

6 The proposed access to the Level 4 lab must receive preliminary approval by the BSL4 Scientific Director.

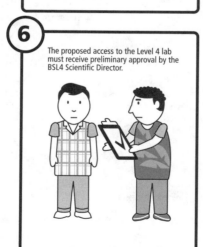

7 The scientist must undergo a rigorous medical examination specifically designed for the BSL4.

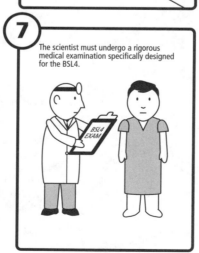

8 The Institutional Biosafety Committee [see "Terms"] must approve the proposed research study.

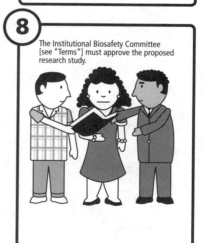

Source: Reproduced from the University of Texas Medical Branch, reprinted with permission from UTMB Public Affairs.

FIGURE 8-5 What a Scientist Must Do to Work in a BSL 4 Laboratory *(Continued)*

9 The scientist must undergo lab-specific orientation and containment-suit training.

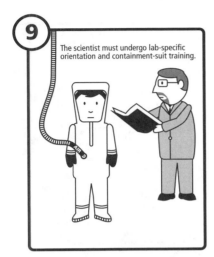

10 Before being considered for solo access to the maximum-containment lab, the scientist must successfully complete at least 100 hours of supervised BSL4 training and log at least 40 entries into the BSL4 lab with a mentor.

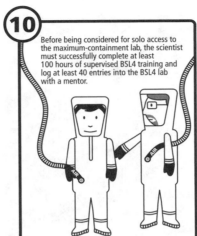

11 Before the scientist is approved for solo access, he or she must obtain written approvals from the BSL4 Scientific Director, the laboratory's Biocontainment Director and the UTMB Biosafety Officer.

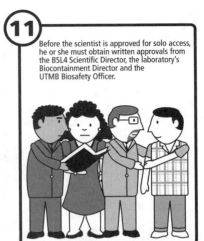

Each time a scientist enters the BSL4 lab:

12 The scientist must pass through a security checkpoint manned 24 hours a day to enter the building. He or she will need electronic and other forms of security clearance to get through a series of locked doors, elevators and stairwells before reaching the first containment door of the BSL4. The trip between the building entrance and the lab entrance is monitored through closed-circuit cameras.

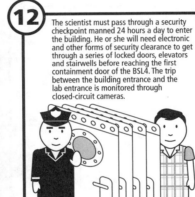

13 The scientist passes through the final locked door to enter the buffer corridor around the laboratory itself. The buffer corridor is under negative pressure so that air flows into the BSL4 area.

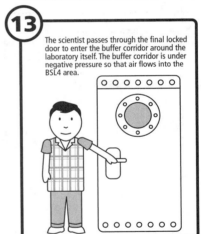

14 From the buffer corridor, the scientist enters a locker room within the BSL4 and changes from street clothes into a jumpsuit.

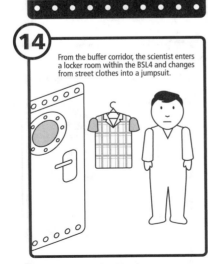

15 The scientist enters the suit room and puts on socks and disposable gloves.

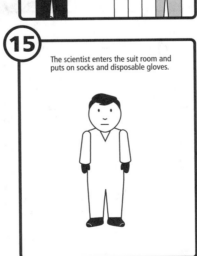

16 The scientist dons a positive-pressure suit to protect him- or herself from any infectious material that might become airborne within the containment lab. Negative air pressure throughout the lab and buffer corridor keeps air flowing into the laboratory to prevent laboratory air from getting out.

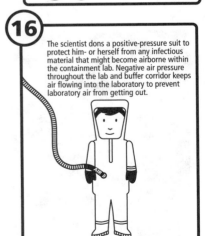

FIGURE 8-5 What a Scientist Must Do to Work in a BSL 4 Laboratory *(Continued)*

17 The scientist passes through an airtight door into the laboratory area.

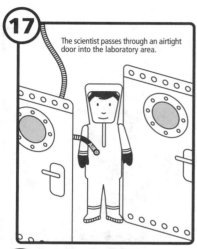

Once inside the lab:

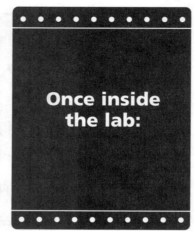

18 The BSL4 laboratory is like a submarine contained in a giant bank vault. Air passes through double HEPA filters to remove any possible airborne materials. Any infectious virus in liquid waste is destroyed by disinfectant and heating at very high temperature.

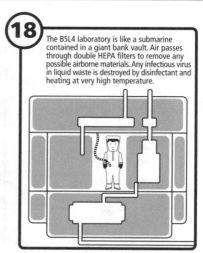

19 The scientist removes a small vial of the agent from a locked freezer.

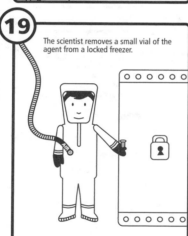

20 The scientist studies the virus under a biosafety cabinet, which uses air pressure, air flow and HEPA filtration to help ensure that no virus particle leaves the biosafety cabinet.

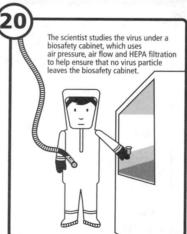

21 When the experiment is complete, the scientist destroys any remaining virus and sterilizes all instruments and surfaces before leaving the laboratory.

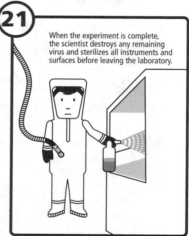

Each time a scientist leaves the BSL4 lab:

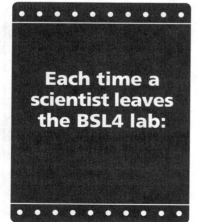

22 He or she exits through a chemical shower that includes a four-minute cycle of disinfectant chemical followed by a four-minute water rinse.

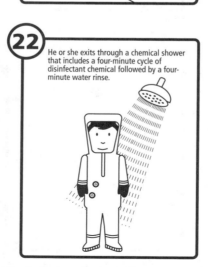

23 The scientist exits the chemical shower into the suit room, and dries and removes the positive-pressure suit. The suit remains in this room.

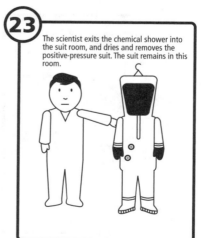

FIGURE 8-5 What a Scientist Must Do to Work in a BSL 4 Laboratory *(Continued)*

24 The scientist removes the jumpsuit and enters a regular shower, where he or she uses soap and shampoo for at least three minutes. Jumpsuits and socks are sterilized before being laundered on-site.

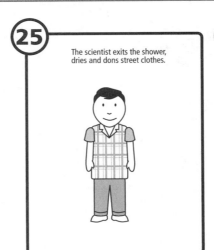

25 The scientist exits the shower, dries and dons street clothes.

26 The scientist exits the locker room into the buffer corridor.

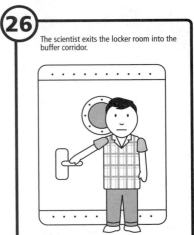

27 The scientist continues through a series of locked doors and exits the building past the security guard at the front door.

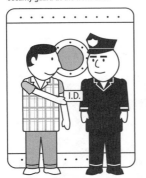

Note: BSL4 labs are closed and decontaminated annually so that systems can be thoroughly checked and maintenance safely performed. In case of a hurricane, the lab is secured and closed.

Terms Used in Containment-Laboratory Work

BIOSAFETY LEVEL 1
Involves work with well-characterized agents not known to cause disease in healthy human adults and that are of minimal potential risk to laboratory personnel or the environment; no special procedures beyond standard laboratory practices are required.

BIOSAFETY LEVEL 2
Involves agents that are of moderate potential hazard for laboratory personnel and the environment (examples: hepatitis A and B, seasonal influenza, HIV). Immunization and/or treatments are available, or the risk of illness or death is extremely low. Some extra precautions, such as the availability of a biosafety cabinet to perform work with infected material, proper receptacles for contaminated needles and sharps, and personal protective equipment (gloves, etc.), are required.

BIOSAFETY LEVEL 3
Involves agents that may cause serious or potentially lethal disease if inhaled (examples: avian influenza, SARS, hantavirus, tuberculosis). Treatments and preventive measures are available against some of these agents, but the rate of infection and risk of complications after exposure is high. This level requires more strict containment measures.

BIOSAFETY LEVEL 4
Involves agents that are highly infectious when inhaled and that cause life-threatening disease in humans and agricultural animals (examples: Ebola, Lassa virus, Nipah virus). Work requires the maximum level of containment in specially designed facilities, as well as extensive training of personnel.

INSTITUTIONAL BIOSAFETY COMMITTEE
Team of microbiologists, infectious disease physicians, safety experts and community members that promotes the safe use and handling of biological agents at UTMB and assures that all activities involving these agents are in compliance with the applicable guidelines, codes and regulations.

SELECT AGENTS
Disease-causing organisms or toxins that have been declared by the federal government to have the potential to pose a severe threat to public health and safety. The Centers for Disease Control and Prevention regulates the laboratories that may possess, use or transfer select agents within the United States.

2/2008

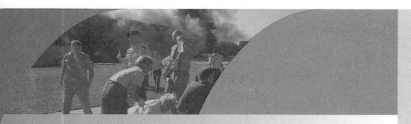

Discussion Questions

1. What are the arguments for keeping or destroying the smallpox virus? Which do you agree with and why?

2. Do we need more or fewer BSL 4 facilities?

3. Would you be comfortable with a BSL 4 facility in your neighborhood? Why or why not?

4. Can you think of ways the private sector might assist in the rapid distribution of medical counter-measures?

5. If you were a delegate to the World Health Assembly, would you vote to destroy or retain smallpox?

REFERENCES

1. U.S. Department of Health and Human Services. Biodefense. National Institute of Allergy and Infectious Diseases. August 10, 2010. Available at: http://www.niaid.nih.gov/topics/BiodefenseRelated/Biodefense/research/Pages/Introduction.aspx. Accessed October 9, 2010.

2. Glowinski IB, Bernstein JB, Kurilla MG. National Institute of Allergy and Infectious Diseases. In: Katz R, Zilinikas R, eds. *Encyclopedia of Bioterrorism Defense*. 2nd ed. New York: Wiley and Sons, May 2011.

3. U.S. Department of Health and Human Services. *Biodefense & Related Programs*. National Institute of Allergy and Infectious Diseases. November 16, 2009. Available at: http://www.niaid.nih.gov/topics/biodefenserelated/pages/default.aspx. Accessed August 23, 2010.

4. Fitch JP. National Biodefense Analysis and Countermeasures Center. In: Katz R, Zilinikas R, eds. *Encyclopedia of Bioterrorism Defense*. 2nd ed. New York: Wiley and Sons, May 2011.

5. U.S. Department of Health and Human Services. Office of Chief Scientist, Integrated Research Facility (OCSIRF). National Institute of Allergy and Infectious Diseases. October 30, 2008. Available at: http://www.niaid.nih.gov/about/organization/dcr/ocsirf/Pages/OCSIFR.aspx. Accessed December 10, 2010.

6. Allen H. Regional Centers of Excellence. In: Katz R, Zilinikas R, eds. *Encyclopedia of Bioterrorism Defense*. 2nd ed. New York: Wiley and Sons, May 2011.

7. Gottron F, Shea DA. CRS Report for Congress: Oversight of High-Containment Biological Laboratories: Issues for Congress. *Federation of American Scientists*. May 4, 2009. Available at: http://www.fas.org/sgp/crs/terror/R40418.pdf. Accessed October 9, 2010.

8. Representative Bart Stupak, Chairman. Committee on Energy and Commerce, Subcommittee on Oversight and Investigations, Hearing on "Federal Oversight of High Containment Bio-Laboratories": Opening Statement. U.S. House of Representatives Committee on Energy and Commerce.

September 22, 2009. Available at: http://democrats.energycommerce.house.gov/Press_111/20090922/stupak_opening.pdf. Accessed October 9, 2010.

9. Takafuji ET. NIAID/NIH Biodefense Research Efforts and Biocontainment Laboratories. *Applied Biosafety*. 2004;9(3):160–163.

10. U.S. Department of Health and Human Services. *National Health Security Strategy of The United States of America*. December 2009. Available at: http://www.phe.gov/Preparedness/planning/authority/nhss/strategy/Documents/nhss-final.pdf. Accessed July 25, 2010.

11. Tucker JB. Developing Medical Countermeasures: From BioShield to BARDA. *Drug Development Research*. June 2009;70(4):224–233.

12. Pandemic and All-Hazards Preparedness Act; Public Law No. 109-417.

13. U.S. Department of Health and Human Services. Public Health Emergency Medical Countermeasures Enterprise (PHEMCE) Management. MedicalCountermeasures.gov. Available at: https://www.medicalcountermeasures.gov/BARDA/PHEMCE/phemce.aspx. Accessed October 9, 2010.

14. Centers for Disease Control and Prevention. Strategic National Stockpile (SNS). *Emergency Preparedness and Response*. May 21, 2010. Available at: http://www.bt.cdc.gov/stockpile/. Accessed October 9, 2010.

15. Courtney B. Study: MedKits Show Promise as a Countermeasure Distribution Strategy. Center for Biosecurity; UPMC. March 14, 2008. Available at: http://www.upmc-biosecurity.org/website/biosecurity_briefing/archive/pub_health_prep/2008-03-14-medkitscntrdiststrategy.html. Accessed October 9, 2010.

16. The White House, Office of the Press Secretary. Executive Order—Medical Countermeasures Following a Biological Attack. December 30, 2009. Available at: http://www.whitehouse.gov/the-press-office/executive-order-medical-countermeasures-following-a-biological-attack. Accessed October 9, 2010.

CHAPTER **9**

International Agreements

LEARNING OBJECTIVES

By the end of this chapter, the reader will be able to:

- Identify the findings of the WMD Prevention Commission.
- Discuss the treaties and international agreements used to prevent the use of weapons of mass destruction (WMD).
- Discuss the international agreements designed to coordinate global response to public health emergencies.
- Evaluate the effectiveness of international agreements in controlling and responding to WMD and other public health emergencies.

INTRODUCTION

In previous chapters, we looked at potential threats to public health from natural, accidental, and intentional events. We have also looked at efforts to enhance public health preparedness through infrastructure development, legislation, and policies and have examined some of the thinking about complicated challenges. Most of these previous chapters, however, have focused on domestic efforts, particularly those efforts of the federal government.

In this chapter, we look at international agreements that have evolved to try to address the threats posed to populations by weapons of mass destruction and infectious diseases. We first look at formal arms control and nonproliferation treaties focused on controlling the use and spread of weapons of mass destruction (WMD). We then examine United Nations Security Council Resolution (UNSCR) 1540 and the World Health Organization (WHO) International Health Regulations (2005).

Recently, policy makers have stressed the need for increased international engagement as a means of preventing

WMD use and ensuring enhanced collaboration in a global response to a public health emergency. The 2010 National Security Strategy reaffirmed America's commitment to using and strengthening the international system (see **Box 9-1**). Policy and guidance have specifically focused on strengthening international regimes related to biological weapons and infectious disease threats.

In December 2008, the Commission on the Prevention of WMD Proliferation and Terrorism released a report called "World at Risk," in which the commission addresses what it believes are the biggest WMD threats and provides

---

BOX 9-1 Importance of International Institutions as Described in the 2010 National Security Strategy

[W]e must focus American engagement on strengthening international institutions and galvanizing the collective action that can serve common interests such as combating violent extremism; stopping the spread of nuclear weapons and securing nuclear materials; achieving balanced and sustainable economic growth; and forging cooperative solutions to the threat of climate change, armed conflict, and pandemic disease.

Source: The White House. *National Security Strategy.* May 2010. Available at: http://www.whitehouse.gov/sites/default/files/rss_viewer/national_security_strategy.pdf. Accessed July 25, 2010.

recommendations for how to mitigate these threats. In this report, the Commission cited biological weapons as the primary threat and strongly recommended reaffirming the importance of international instruments, including the Biological Weapons Convention (BWC) and the International Health Regulations (2005).[1] Likewise, the 2009 National Strategy for Countering Biological Threats calls for the revitalization of the BWC and integrating efforts to meet international obligations that lie at the nexus of security, health, and science.[2] Despite real and perceived challenges associated with international regimes, they are a useful tool in addressing global challenges, and the United States appears to be committed to strengthening and utilizing international instruments.

EARLY AGREEMENTS

There have been a series of international agreements about security and weapons of war aimed at addressing what we now term weapons of mass destruction. On April 24, 1863, the U.S. War Department issued General Orders 100, which declared "The use of poison in any manner, be it to poison wells, or foods, or arms, is wholly excluded from modern warfare."[3](Sec. III, number 70) Thirty-plus years later, the 1899 Hague Convention (II) declared "it is especially prohibited … [t]o employ poison or poisoned arms."[4](Sec. 2, Chap. 3, Art. 23)

The 1907 Hague Convention repeated this same text,[5] and it was not until 1925 that the first agreement on chemical and biological weapons was signed that is still considered applicable under customary international law. On June 17, 1925, 38 nations signed the Geneva Protocol for the Prohibition of the Use in War of Asphyxiating, Poisonous or Other Gasses, and of Bacteriological Methods of Warfare, known as the Geneva Protocol, the text of which is reproduced in **Box 9-2**. (The United States signed the Geneva Protocol but did not ratify it until 1975.) This agreement, developed in the aftermath of wide-scale chemical weapons use during World War I, does not ban the possession of chemical or biological weapons (CBW) but prohibits using them in war. In actuality, this is a "no first use" agreement; that is, many nations interpreted it to mean that they would not use CBW in war, but if used against a nation, they would—and could—retaliate in kind.

CHEMICAL WEAPONS CONVENTION

The Chemical Weapons Convention (CWC) was concluded in 1993 and entered into force in 1997. As of December 2010, there were 188 parties, with two additional signatories (Israel and Myanmar) that had yet to ratify the agreement. Building on the Geneva Protocol, the CWC explicitly prohibits the use of chemical weapons and bans the development, production, stockpile, and transfer of such agents. Under the agreement,

states are required to declare any past chemical weapons program that existed after January 1, 1946, and obligates states that had chemical weapons to destroy their stockpiles within 10 years. The destruction of chemical weapons is a complicated and expensive endeavor, and this total destruction has not yet been completed. Of the 71,194 metric tons of chemical agents that have been declared by states, 60.58% has been destroyed, and only 45.56% of the chemical munitions and containers have been destroyed as of 2010.[6] The time line for destruction has been extended to 2012, but it is clear that all declared agents, munitions, and containers will not be destroyed by this deadline.

The CWC established the Organization for the Prohibition of Chemical Weapons (OPCW), based in The Hague, which conducts inspections, ensures compliance with the treaty, and provides a forum for cooperation and consultation.

THE NUCLEAR NONPROLIFERATION TREATY

The Treaty on the Nonproliferation of Nuclear Weapons (known as the Nuclear Nonproliferation Treaty, or NPT) was signed in 1968 and entered into force in March 1970. There are 189 signatories, 5 of whom are known to have nuclear weapons (the United States, United Kingdom, France, Russia, and China). Four nations known or suspected of having or wanting nuclear weapons are not signatories: India, Pakistan, Israel, and North Korea (which withdrew from the treaty in 2003).

The purpose of the NPT is to limit the spread of nuclear weapons, encourage disarmament, and foster the right to peacefully use nuclear technology. While acknowledging that nations have nuclear weapons, the purpose of this treaty is to keep these weapons from spreading into the hands of other nations and to make certain that nations with the knowledge to build such weapons refrain from doing so.

UNITED NATIONS SECURITY COUNCIL RESOLUTION 1540

In 2004, the United Nations Security Council adopted Resolution 1540, obligating UN member-states to ensure they do not support nonstate actors in their efforts to develop, acquire, possess, or use nuclear, chemical, or biological weapons. To do this, the resolution obligates states to create or modify domestic legislation to criminalize the proliferation or use of WMD by nonstate actors. Not only must countries have appropriate legislation in place, but there must also be a means to enforce the legislation to prevent proliferation and use of chemical, biological, or nuclear weapons.

UNSCR 1540 is designed to complement other international regimes. The NPT and the International Atomic Energy Association (IAEA) have programs supportive of Resolu-

BOX 9-2 Geneva Protocol

Protocol for the Prohibition of the Use in War of Asphyxiating, Poisonous or other Gases, and of Bacteriological Methods of Warfare. Signed at Geneva, June 17, 1925.

THE UNDERSIGNED PLENIPOTENTIARIES, in the name of their respective Governments :

Whereas the use in war of asphyxiating, poisonous or other gases, and of all analogous liquids, materials or devices, has been justly condemned by the general opinion of the civilised world; and

Whereas the prohibition of such use has been declared in Treaties to which the majority of Powers of the world are Parties; and

To the end that this prohibition shall be universally accepted as a part of International Law, binding alike the conscience and the practice of nations;

DECLARE:

That the High Contracting Parties, so far as they are not already Parties to Treaties prohibiting such use, accept this prohibition, agree to extend this prohibition to the use of bacteriological methods of warfare and agree to be bound as between themselves according to the terms of this declaration.

The High Contracting Parties will exert every effort to induce other States to accede to the present Protocol. Such accession will be notified to the Government of the French Republic, and by the latter to all signatory and acceding Powers, and will take effect on the date of the notification by the Government of the French Republic.

The present Protocol, of which the French and English texts are both authentic, shall be ratified as soon as possible. It shall bear today's date.

The ratifications of the present Protocol shall be addressed to the Government of the French Republic, which will at once notify the deposit of such ratification to each of the signatory and acceding Powers.

The instruments of ratification of and accession to the present Protocol will remain deposited in the archives of the Government of the French Republic.

The present Protocol will come into force for each signatory Power as from the date of deposit of its ratification, and, from that moment, each Power will be bound as regards other Powers which have already deposited their ratifications.

Source: United Nations. *Protocol for the Prohibition of the Use in War of Asphyxiating, Poisonous or Other Gases, and of Bacteriological Methods of Warfare.* June 17, 1925. Available at: http://www.un.org/disarmament/WMD/Bio/pdf/Status_Protocol.pdf. Accessed October 9, 2010.

tion 1540, including providing legislative and technical assistance. The resolution is also in line with CWC obligations and OPCW action plans. A 1540 Committee, established by the Resolution, monitors global implementation, which contributes to compliance assessments of the BWC.

AUSTRALIA GROUP

While not a formal international agreement, there is an informal group of countries (and the European Commission) known as the Australia Group. Established in 1985, this group creates a list of items it believes has the potential to help "would-be proliferators" develop or acquire chemical or biological weapons.[7] Those items are then subject to export con-

trols. While this group's efforts are not legally binding, they are supportive of obligations under the BWC and CWC.

BIOLOGICAL WEAPONS CONVENTION

In 1972, nations around the world agreed to the Biological and Toxin Weapons Convention (BWC). To date, 164 nations have become party to the agreement, with an additional 13 that have signed but not yet ratified. Under the BWC, nations agree never to develop, produce, stockpile, acquire, or retain any biological agent for other than peaceful purposes. The agreement also obliges parties to facilitate the exchange of equipment, materials, and information related to biological agents for peaceful purposes.

The BWC consists of a preamble and 12 articles, described here:[8]

- **Preamble:** Cites the Geneva Protocol and reaffirms adherence to those principles, in essence pointing to the previous agreement not to use biological weapons, stating that such use would "be repugnant to the conscience of mankind."
- **Article I:** Never in any circumstances should a state develop, produce, stockpile, or otherwise acquire or retain biological agents or toxins, or weapons, equipment, or means to deliver such agents for hostile purposes.
- **Article II:** If a state has such agents or toxins, they must be destroyed immediately or diverted for peaceful purposes.
- **Article III:** No state will transfer, assist, encourage, or induce any other state or entity to manufacture or acquire any agent, toxin, weapons, or delivery mechanisms.
- **Article IV:** Each state must take necessary measures to prohibit and prevent the development, acquisition, or retention of biological agents or toxins or delivery mechanisms in all areas under its jurisdiction.
- **Article V:** All states parties must work with each other to solve any problems associated with the agreement and can use appropriate international procedures.
- **Article VI:** If a state finds another state to be in breach of its obligations under the BWC, the state can lodge a complaint with the United Nations Security Council. States should cooperate with the Security Council if it wishes to carry out an investigation.
- **Article VII:** States will provide assistance and support to a nation that requests aid as a result of being exposed to danger per a violation of the BWC.
- **Article VIII:** Nothing in the BWC should be interpreted as limiting or detracting from the Geneva Protocol.
- **Article IX:** Each state recognizes the importance of prohibiting chemical weapons use and agrees to negotiate to reach a separate agreement on chemical weapons. (Note: The CWC came about almost 20 years after the BWC.)
- **Article X:** The right of states' parties to participate in the peaceful exchange of equipment, material, and technology related to biological and toxin agents is reaffirmed. Here, it declares that parties with resources should help those with less.
- **Article XI, XII, XIII** are procedural articles regarding amendments, entry into force, duration, and ratification.

Unlike the CWC, the BWC does not have a verification mechanism—meaning there is no means under the treaty for countries to inspect and verify that another nation is either compliant with or in violation of its treaty obligations. During the 1990s, such a mechanisms were proposed, debated, and negotiated. In 2001, however, after almost a decade of discussion, the United States pulled out, stating that advances in technology and other factors made the BWC virtually unverifiable, and therefore, the proposed mechanisms would not be effective. With the departure of the United States from the negotiations, the verification protocol was dropped. The United States, however, remained committed to the BWC and proposed what was called a "work program," in which states' parties meet each year to discuss topics relevant to the BWC, using the treaty as a forum for sharing ideas, forming collaborations, and advancing knowledge on a range of topics. This program was adopted and has since been used to discuss biosecurity, codes of conduct, disease surveillance, technology transfer, investigating allegations of use, and a variety of topics directly related to the BWC.

INTERNATIONAL HEALTH REGULATIONS (2005)

In 2005, after almost a decade of negotiations, the World Health Assembly (WHA) of the WHO adopted the International Health Regulations [IHR (2005)]. This agreement, binding on all member-states of the WHA, revises previous international agreements, going back to 1891, which focused on international cooperation for containing a short, finite list of historically relevant diseases. The updated version of the regulations recognizes the threat of emerging infectious diseases; the globalization of society; and the need for improved surveillance, response, communication, and coordination to effectively detect and respond to public health threats (see **Table 9-1**).

IHR (2005) includes some major changes to the international regime for controlling communicable diseases. First, this version of the IHR addresses anything that may constitute a public health emergency of international concern (PHEIC). A PHEIC is defined using a decision-making algorithm to determine if an event is unusual or unexpected, if the public health impact is serious, if there is a significant risk of international spread, and if the event might require travel and trade restrictions.[9(Annex 2)] It requires countries to identify and report any potential PHEIC in a timely fashion to the WHO and provides for an effective response through evidence-based recommendations, assistance, transparency, and communication. Countries are obligated to develop basic core competencies for disease surveillance and response and to have a focal point in place for communication to and from the WHO.

TABLE 9-1 Evolution of the International Health Regulations, 1951 to the Present

IHR Component	1951–2007	2007–Present
Type of Threats	Cholera, Plague, Yellow Fever, and Smallpox (removed after eradication)	Public Health Emergency of International Concern
Focus	Control of disease at ports and borders	Detect, report, and contain public health threats at ports, borders, and anywhere they might occur to prevent international spread
Communication	Countries fax reports to WHO; nations identify authorities on an ad hoc basis	Notifications to and from WHO via IHR national focal points (NFP) and WHO's secure website
Notification	Report to WHO within 24 hours	Report to WHO within 24. 72 hours to respond to follow up requests
Coordinated Response	No mechanism for coordinating international response to contain disease. Predetermined public health controls at borders and ports	WHO Assistance in response and provision of recommended measures using best available evidence
National Capacity	Public health and infection control at ports of entry	Capacity to detect, assess, report, and respond to public health threats at the national and local levels

Source: Modified from Fischer J, Katz R. International Health Regulations 101, Stimson Center. IHR (2005): from the global to the local, March 2010. Available at www.stimson.org/ihr/

A primary purpose of IHR (2005) is to improve global health security through international collaboration and communication to detect and contain public health emergencies at the source. Full implementation requires multisectoral engagement and resources. Countries have until 2012 to become compliant with IHR (2005), although it is clear that some countries will require additional time to build the necessary public health infrastructure to meet core capacities for surveillance and response. IHR (2005) was tested for the first time during the 2009–2010 H1N1 influenza pandemic, and overall, the international framework created by the regulations greatly assisted in enabling the WHO to be notified of the virus in a timely fashion, coordinate response to nations who needed assistance, and communicate evidence-based recommendations globally.

THE FUNCTIONALITY OF INTERNATIONAL AGREEMENTS

Some argue that international agreements are not a good way to force nations to act a particular way, to promote an agenda, or to facilitate cooperation. This argument is based on the concept that nations are sovereign states, and regardless of what document they may have signed, they will do whatever they see as in their national interests. Because of this concern, many agreements have associated penalties for violations. In some cases, those violations may be official United Nations

sanctions, with economic and political consequences. In other cases, the enforcement mechanism may be less formal, such as travel and trade recommendations made by the WHO that might result in economic losses for a noncompliant country.

Even in the absence of an enforcement mechanism, it can be argued that international agreements are vital tools in preparedness and prevention. They create an important forum for international dialogue, for information exchange, and for addressing serious global challenges. In some cases, this dialogue may be at a very high political level, and in other cases these fora become opportunities for pragmatic cooperation leading to measurable changes.

While perceptions of the importance of international agreements may vary, it is clear that they are important tools both internationally and domestically in shaping policy and global interactions.

KEY WORDS

International agreements
Biological Weapons Convention
Chemical Weapons Convention
Nuclear Nonproliferation Treaty
Geneva Protocol
Australia Group
UNSCR 1540
International Health Regulations

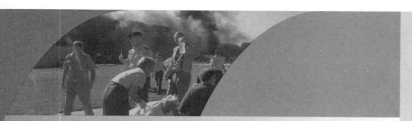

Discussion Questions

1. What are the major differences among the Geneva Protocol, the BWC, and the CWC?

2. Should all international agreements have enforcement mechanisms? Should IHR (2005) have an enforcement mechanism?

3. In your opinion, are international agreements useful? Why or why not? Can you provide an example of where an agreement has served as a useful tool for addressing an event? Can you provide an example of where an agreement did not serve its intended purpose?

4. Does the international community require a new treaty for public health preparedness? If so, what would it say?

REFERENCES

1. Graham B, Talent J, Allison G, et al. *World at Risk: The Report of the Commission on the Prevention of WMD Proliferation and Terrorism.* December 2008. Available at: http://www.absa.org/leg/WorldAtRisk.pdf. Accessed July 10, 2010.

2. National Security Council. National Strategy for Countering Biological Threats. The White House. November 2009. Available at: http://www.whitehouse.gov/sites/default/files/National_Strategy_for_Countering_BioThreats.pdf. Accessed September 10, 2010.

3. U.S. War Department. Lieber Code of 1863; General Orders No. 100. U.S. Air Force, Air University. 1863. Available at: http://www.au.af.mil/au/awc/awcgate/law/liebercode.htm. Accessed October 9, 2010.

4. Convention (II) with Respect to the Laws and Customs of War on Land and Its Annex: Regulations Concerning the Laws and Customs of War on Land. The Biological and Toxin Weapons Convention Website. July 29, 1899. Available at: http://www.opbw.org/int_inst/sec_docs/1899HC-TEXT.pdf. Accessed October 9, 2010.

5. Convention (IV) Respecting the Laws and Customs of War on Land and Its Annex: Regulations Concerning the Laws and Customs of War on Land. International Committee of the Red Cross. October 18, 1907. Available at: http://www.icrc.org/ihl.nsf/FULL/195?OpenDocument. Accessed October 9, 2010.

6. Organisation for the Prohibition of Chemical Weapons. *Demilitarisation: Latest Facts and Figures.* July 31, 2010. Available at: http://www.opcw.org/our-work/demilitarisation/. Accessed October 9, 2010.

7. The Australia Group. Available at: http://www.australiagroup.net/en/index.html. Accessed October 9, 2010.

8. Convention on the Prohibition of the Development, Production and Stockpiling of Bacteriological (Biological) and Toxin Weapons and on Their Destruction. Available at: http://www.unog.ch/80256EDD006B8954/(httpAssets)/C4048678A93B6934C1257188004848D0/$file/BWC-text-English.pdf. Accessed December 10, 2010.

9. World Health Organization. International Health Regulations (2005), 2nd ed. 2008. Available at: http://whqlibdoc.who.int/publications/2008/9789241580410_eng.pdf. Accessed May 23, 2011

Attribution and Investigations

INTRODUCTION

Responding to and investigating disease outbreaks and public health events is a core component of the public health mission. Basic training in epidemiology outlines the steps public health professionals take in a disease outbreak: determine the existence of an outbreak; confirm the diagnosis; define a case; count cases; identify person, place, and time (the who, what, and when of the event); determine who is at risk of becoming ill; develop and test hypotheses regarding exposure; and contain the outbreak to minimize morbidity and mortality in the population. Epidemiologists are trained to conduct these investigations. They know how to determine if an epidemic is taking place; they work with the public health laboratories to examine specimens; they identify possible and probable cases; they coordinate with the medical system to appropriately treat patients; they analyze data to determine causation; they use all of the resources available to them to contain and mitigate the consequences of the event.

But what happens when a disease outbreak or public health emergency is suspected of being an intentional event? And can public health officials anticipate and plan for such an event?

In this chapter we will look at how one begins to differentiate between naturally occurring events and intentional events and, if an event is suspected of being intentional, what steps must be taken to minimize the damages incurred. The investigation can suddenly become much more complicated and involve many new players. We will look at some of the work that has been done to build relationships among the organizations that need to work together on these types of investigations.

DIFFERENTIATING BETWEEN NATURAL AND INTENTIONAL EVENTS

One of the ways in which biological agents can be effective weapons is through plausible deniability—they can be extremely difficult to detect. In fact, it can almost be impossible to differentiate between a naturally occurring disease and an intentional event. Of course, this is not always the case. A cluster of smallpox cases outside of the two designated smallpox repository laboratories would automatically be considered an intentional event until proven otherwise because smallpox is no longer circulating naturally. A large explosion releasing a visible cloud of agents resulting in population morbidity and mortality would most certainly be investigated as an intentional event. Other outbreaks, though, are more complicated. Several researchers have tried to identify and characterize the epidemiology of an intentional event to provide clues that something might not be of natural origin.[1,2,3] Their collective findings include the following:

- Intentional events are more likely to have a point source. This means that individuals are exposed to the agent during one time period so that infected individuals begin to show symptoms at about the same time. The epidemic curve for a point source event usually has a sharp rise in cases at one time, with most cases developing within a short time period. (See **Figure 10-1**.)
- An intentional event may involve a larger-than-expected number of cases.
- The disease may be more severe than expected from a naturally occurring event.
- There may be unusual routes of exposure (e.g., airborne as opposed to gastrointestinal).
- The disease may be unusual for a given geographic area.
- The outbreak may involve an unusual strain or variant of an agent.
- There may be distinctly higher attack rates in individuals exposed to the agent during specific times or in specific areas.
- Simultaneous morbidity and mortality in animals may signal an airborne release of an agent.
- There may be corroborating intelligence information suggesting intent by an actor to use biological agents.

Regardless of whether the event is naturally occurring or intentional (or even accidental), it will still start with detection through surveillance mechanisms, followed by an investigation. The public health community will need to detect, identify, and characterize the event and respond through treatment and containment. If the event is not naturally occurring, there will also need to be an attribution assessment to determine the source of the agent and the perpetrator(s) of the attack.

ATTRIBUTION ASSESSMENTS

While the public health community is responsible for detecting, identifying, and responding to an intentional-use event to safeguard population health, law enforcement officials and policy makers are responsible for determining and verifying the origin or source, sponsorship, delivery, and responsible party associated with an intentional-use event. The task of answering "Who did it?" is called an attribution assessment. This assessment may be used for a variety of purposes, ranging from criminal prosecution of individuals to diplomatic actions against nations. The strength of the evidence necessary for the attribution assessment, however, may vary depending on the intended use; strong evidence may be used in a court of law, while weaker evidence may be used to spark diplomatic actions.

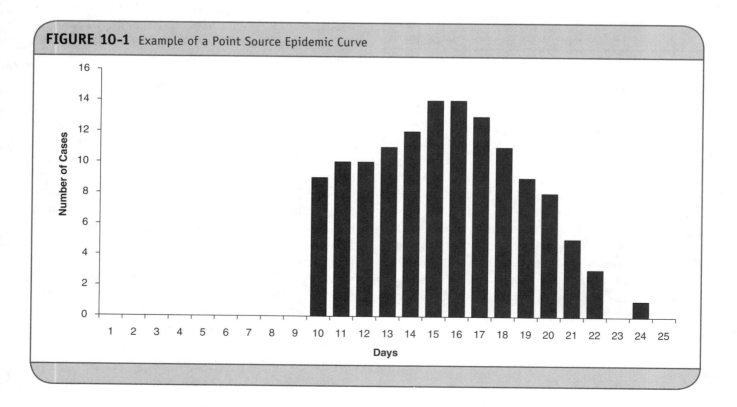

FIGURE 10-1 Example of a Point Source Epidemic Curve

To make an attribution assessment, investigators need to link the agent used in an event to a source and to a specified perpetrator. They need to identify if a crime occurred and, if so, what exactly happened, when, and why. They need to determine what evidence is necessary to answer these questions.[4] Depending on the evidence and the event, microbial forensics may need to be used. *Microbial forensics* is the application of both forensic science and molecular epidemiology to problems involving biological agents.[5] It employs themes and concepts from these disciplines to determine the molecular identity of the agent if it can be linked to a source and, if so, how precisely it can be linked. Depending on the availability of source data, microbial forensics may provide useful data that can be used during a criminal prosecution or possibly an investigative lead that can assist in the larger attribution investigation.

DOMESTIC INVESTIGATIONS OF SUSPECTED BIOLOGICAL WEAPONS USE

As discussed, the first indication that a potential intentional-use event has occurred will likely come from the local public health surveillance systems. That event is then reported to state and possibly federal authorities while, at the same time, public health officials begin to investigate the event. At the first indication that the event may be intentional, law enforcement personnel become involved. Law enforcement personnel then engage in the process of evidence collection, ensuring chain of custody of evidence is maintained so that it can be introduced at trials, delivering biological samples to specific laboratories in the Laboratory Response Network (LRN) to ensure proper analysis, obtaining original documents when appropriate, and taking witness statements regarding the event.

In the past, law enforcement and public health often conducted their investigations separately. The National Response Framework's Biological Incident Annex provided guidance for which agency had lead for particular aspects of the investigation (see **Table 10-1**), but there was limited collaboration, information sharing, and a lot of getting in each others' way. Recent efforts, however, on the part of both the FBI and the CDC have produced protocols and best practices for joint criminal and epidemiological investigations (known as Crim-Epi). These agencies jointly produce a handbook for investigators outlining legal authorities, roles and responsibilities, information exchanges, and how to conduct joint interviews.[6] Not only are the FBI and CDC now coordinating and collaborating on investigations to identify agents, prevent the spread of disease, and apprehend those responsible, they conduct training for local entities, as well as for other countries.[7]

By far the most famous domestic investigation of an alleged BW incident was the anthrax letters of 2001—an investigation known as "Amerithrax." This case is described in **Box 10-1**.

INTERNATIONAL INVESTIGATIONS OF SUSPECTED BIOLOGICAL WEAPONS USE

International investigations of suspected intentional-use events, like those in the domestic arena, start with a local public health system detecting that something out of the ordinary in kind or scope has happened. In some cases, these first reports may come from nongovernmental organizations, particularly if the reports are from refugee camps or remote populations. The event is then reported to the national-level authorities, and, depending on the type of event, it may be reported to either the World Health Organization or the United Nations.

Under the International Health Regulations (2005), states parties must notify the WHO of any event that may constitute a public health emergency of international concern (PHEIC). These include events that are unusual or unexpected in nature, including those of unknown causes or sources. In the case of an intentional—or suspected intentional—use event, the state would notify the WHO. The WHO would then offer assistance to respond to the event, often through the Global Outbreak Alert and Response Network (GOARN). GOARN was established in 1997 and formalized in 2000. It is a network of public health and medical professionals, laboratorians, and institutions that partner to investigate, respond to, and contain disease outbreaks. According to the WHO, GOARN aims to detect, verify, and contain epidemics and, specifically, intentional releases of biological agents.[8]

Not only does the WHO have investigative and response teams through GOARN, but they also partner with other international organizations, such as the Food and Agriculture Organization (FAO) of the UN and the World Organization of Animal Health (OIE), both of which may investigate disease outbreaks in animals.

When a country suspects that there has been an intentional use of biological or chemical weapons, the country can make a request to the UN Secretary General to formally investigate the allegations. The UN General Assembly and the Security Council established a mandate through multiple resolutions (including Resolution 620 in 1988, and 42/37C) for the Secretary General (SG) to carry on chemical and biological weapons (CBW) use investigations. (This mandate is known as the UN Secretary General's Mechanism.) While it applies to both biological weapons (BW) and chemical weapons (CW), the Organization for the Prohibition of Chemical Weapons

TABLE 10-1 National Response Framework: Biological Incident Annex

Element of Biological Incident Response	Federal Agencies—Lead
Rapid detection of the outbreak or introduction of a biological agent into the environment.	DHHS (humans); USDA (animals); Department of Interior (wildlife); DHS (National Biosurveillance Integration Center)
Rapid dissemination of key safety information, appropriate personal protective equipment, and necessary medical precautions.	DHHS
Swift agent identification and confirmation.	DHHS, FBI (Laboratory Response Network and Food Emergency Response Network)
Identification of the population at risk (to include animals, marine life, and plants).	DHHS (humans); USDA (animals and plants); Department of Interior (wildlife)
Determination of how the agent is transmitted, including an assessment of the efficiency of transmission.	DHHS
Determination of susceptibility to prophylaxis and treatment.	DHHS
Definition of the public health and medical services, human services, and mental health implications.	DHHS
Control and containment of the epidemic when possible and use of mitigation strategies when containment is not possible (e.g., in the event of an influenza pandemic).	DHHS
Identification of the law enforcement implications/assessment of the threat.	FBI
Augmentation and surging of local health and medical resources.	DHHS
Protection of the population through appropriate public health and medical actions.	DHHS
Dissemination of information to enlist public support and provide risk communication assistance to responsible authorities.	DHHS, DHS
Assessment of environmental contamination and cleanup/decontamination/proper disposal of bioagents that persist in the environment and provision of consultation on the safety of drinking water and food products that may be derived from directly or environmentally exposed animals, crops, plants and trees, or marine life.	EPA
Tracking and preventing secondary or additional disease outbreak.	DHHS
Administration of countermeasures when appropriate.	DHHS

Notes:
DHHS is in charge of overall preparation and response
If incident response requires multiagency participation, DHS serves as incident coordinator
Source: FEMA. *Biological Incident Annex.* August 2008. Available at: http://www.fema.gov/pdf/emergency/nrf/nrf_BiologicalIncidentAnnex.pdf. Accessed August 23, 2010.

(OPCW) now has the ability to investigate CW investigations, so the mechanism is now primarily relevant for BW.

The Secretary General's mechanism allows any member state to submit a report of alleged use to the Secretary General. The Secretary General can then decide to launch an investigation utilizing a team of qualified experts, provided by the member states. The investigation, however, can only operate in countries that have provided express permission.

The mechanism was used a dozen times starting in the early 1980s, with the last investigations occurring in 1992.[9]

One of the challenges of the Secretary General's Mechanism was that it is difficult to get experts on the ground to conduct an investigation in a timely fashion. Thus, attempts to determine the facts of a case are complicated by time delays and inability to access evidence. Recently, the UN signed a memorandum of understanding (MOU) with the WHO that

BOX 10-1 Amerithrax Case Study

In the weeks following the September 11, 2001, attacks, several letters containing anthrax were mailed to news outlets and U.S. senators. The letters contained white powder and a cursory note. The letter sent to Senator Leahy read, "YOU CAN NOT STOP US. WE HAVE THIS ANTHRAX. YOU DIE NOW. ARE YOU AFRAID? DEATH TO AMERICA. DEATH TO ISRAEL. ALLAH IS GREAT." The letters led to 22 cases of anthrax, five deaths, large-scale decontamination efforts, and what amounted to a seven-year investigation by the FBI and U.S. Postal Service inspectors.

Massive amounts of evidence were collected during the investigation, but investigators were limited by the scientific methods available to them. Over the course of the investigation, new methods in microbial forensics were developed to eventually trace the anthrax sent in the letters to a single spore-batch of anthrax. The final determination of the perpetrator required a combination of traditional law enforcement methods with new methods of scientific analysis.

In the end, the investigation led to Dr. Bruce Ivins, an employee at USAMRIID at Fort Detrick. Dr. Ivins committed suicide in July 2008 before he could formally be indicted.

Amerithrax by the Numbers:

- At least 5 letters sent in September and October 2001.
- 22 cases of anthrax.
- 5 dead from anthrax.
- Another 31 tested positive for exposure but did not become ill.
- 10,000 "at-risk" individuals underwent antibiotic prophylaxis.
- 35 postal facilities and mailrooms contaminated.
- Anthrax detected in 7 buildings on Capitol Hill.
- From October through December 2001, the LRN tested more than 120,000 clinical and environmental samples.
- 7-year investigation.
- 600,000 investigator work-hours.
- 10,000 witness interviews.
- 80 searchers.
- 6,000 items of potential evidence.
- 5,730 samples collected from 60 sites.
- Cooperation from 29 government, university, and commercial labs.
- Amerithrax task force staffed by 25–30 full-time investigators.
- 5,750 grand jury subpoenas.
- 1,000 possible suspects.
- 1 perpetrator, never tried for the crime.

Source: U.S. Department of Justice. *Amerithrax Investigative Summary*. February 19, 2010. Available at: http://www.justice.gov/amerithrax/docs/amx-investigative-summary.pdf. Accessed December 10, 2010.

will allow the WHO to share information and resources, including data collected during its own investigations, with UN fact-finding teams.[10]

In addition to the UN Secretary General's Mechanism, the GOARN, and the other international organizations involved in alleged use investigations, there are many national and regional entities that would/could become involved in investigations, each bringing its own expertise to the situation. The North American Treaty Organization (NATO), for example, has a Multinational CBRN Defense Battalion that can provide response teams, laboratory assets, and logistical support while investigating allegations of CBW use in NATO countries. The European Union Center for Disease Prevention and Control (ECDC) has a unit for responding to outbreaks and other health threats of unknown origin. Interpol and Europol both support law enforcement officials in the field, providing a resource for national-level law enforcement efforts in response to an alleged intentional-use event.[11] Finally, in most cases, outbreak investigations and alleged use investigations will be led by the national entity. Depending on the resources available to that country, there may be assistance from any of the previously mentioned organizations.

SUMMARY

It is evident that responding to public health emergencies to protect population health is complicated. Responding to public health emergencies with the goal of protecting population health, as well as determining if the event was intentional and, if so, who committed the crime, in a manner that will provide strong enough evidence to bring a perpetrator to justice or influence foreign policy decisions is even more complicated. Many entities need to become involved, not all of which have the same goals, but many of which need to use the same data. Collaboration among law enforcement, security, and public health entities greatly strengthens the ability of all sectors to do their jobs well.

KEY WORDS

Outbreak investigation
Attribution assessment
Microbial forensics
Crim-Epi
Global Outbreak Alert Response Network
Amerithrax

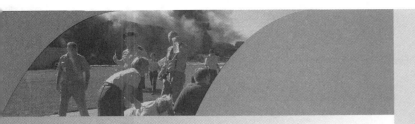

Discussion Questions

1. If faced with a suspicious disease outbreak, what questions would you ask to begin to determine if the event was natural, intentional, or accidental?

2. What organizations would you work with to make the preceding determination?

3. What could/should be improved to make accurate and timely attribution assessments?

4. What kind of cooperation do you think would be necessary to have a complete international investigation of an alleged CBW use event?

REFERENCES

1. Pavlin JA. Epidemiology of Bioterrorism. *Emerging Infectious Diseases*. July–August 1999;5(4):528–530.

2. Khan AS, Morse S, Lillibridge S. Public-Health Preparedness for Biological Terrorism in the USA. *The Lancet*. September 2000;356(9236):1179–1182.

3. Dembek ZF, Kortepeter MG, Pavlin JA. Discernment between Deliberate and Natural Infectious Disease Outbreaks. *Epidemiology and Infection*. April 2007;135(3):353–371.

4. Bahr E. Attribution of Biological Weapons Use. In: Katz R, Zilinikas R, eds. *Encyclopedia of Bioterrorism Defense*. 2nd ed. New York: Wiley and Sons, May 2011.

5. Budowle B, Burans JP, Breeze RG, Wilson MR, Chakraborty R. Microbial Forensics. In: Budowle B, Schutzer SE, Breeze RG, eds. *Microbial Forensics*. Elsevier Academic Press, 2005.

6. Centers for Disease Control and Prevention. *Criminal and Epidemiological Investigation Handbook*. Available at: http://www2.cdc.gov/phlp/ForensicEpi/docs/Crim_Epi_Hdbk.pdf. Accessed November 5, 2010.

7. U.S. Government. *Joint Public Health and Law Enforcement Investigations: Enhancing Relationships to Improve Readiness*. Geneva, Switzerland: Meeting of the States Parties to the Convention on the Prohibition of the Development, Production and Stockpiling of Bacteriological (Biological) and Toxin Weapons and on Their Destruction. August 12, 2010.

8. World Health Organization. *Global Alert and Response (GAR): Alert & Response Operations*. Available at: http://www.who.int/csr/alertresponse/en/. Accessed November 5, 2010.

9. Smidovich N. *The Secretary-General's Investigations of Alleged Use of Chemical, Biological or Toxin Weapons*. The United Nations Office at Geneva. August 25, 2010. Available at: http://www.unog.ch/__80256ee600585943.nsf/%28httpPages%29/792fa92b5d9f75c6c12577c000514299?OpenDocument&ExpandSection=5#_Section5. Accessed November 5, 2010.

10. Implementation Support Unit. *The Role of International Organizations in the Provision of Assistance and Coordination in the Case of Alleged Use of Biological or Toxin Weapons*. Geneva: Meeting of the States Parties to the Convention on the Prohibition of the Development, Production and Stockpiling of Bacteriological (Biological) and Toxin Weapons and on Their Destruction. August 5, 2010.

11. Commission of the European Communities. Bridging Security and Health: Towards the Identification of Good Practices in the Response to CBRN Incidents and the Security of CBR Substances. Available at: http://ec.europa.eu/health/ph_threats/com/preparedness/docs/bridging_en.pdf. Accessed November 5, 2010.

Surveillance

INTRODUCTION

One of the most effective tools for public health preparedness is a comprehensive disease surveillance system. Comprehensive biosurveillance allows for the rapid detection, identification, characterization, and containment of biological threats. This capability is essential to the health of populations, effective biodefense, and national security. An effective biosurveillance capability is thus essential for preparedness, detection, and response to biological outbreaks.

In this chapter, we describe the current system for biosurveillance, the policy guidance documents supporting the development of this capacity, and the multitude of surveillance tools currently being utilized for detection of potential biological threats and other public health emergencies. The links between domestic and global surveillance systems will also be examined.

Biosurveillance can be defined as any method to detect and monitor a biological incident whether of intentional or natural origin. Homeland Security Presidential Directive 21 (HSPD-21) defines biosurveillance as "the process of active data-gathering with appropriate analysis and interpretation of biosphere data that might relate to disease activity and threats to human or animal health—whether infectious, toxic, metabolic, or otherwise, and regardless of intentional or natural origin—in order to achieve early warning of health threats, early detection of health events, and overall situational awareness of disease activity."[1] This notion of situational awareness is defined as the basic ability to understand what is going on in a given area. It is the ability to collect and analyze data in order to make appropriately informed predictions and decisions. A more recent definition of biosurveillance is discussed in **Box 11-1**.

Disease surveillance as a concept has evolved from the observation of individuals suspected of being ill[2] to the current conception of ongoing, systematic collection, analysis, and reporting of health-related data.[3] The purpose of these activities is to monitor disease and population health and detect abnormal events. Understanding the baseline health conditions of a population allows decision makers to set priorities, design research programs, and identify short- and long-term public health risks. Being able to detect an abnormality, an unusual health threat, an emerging infectious disease, or any other potential public health emergency allows for a quick and effective response to treat patients, contain the spread of disease, and mitigate the consequences of the event. (See **Figure 11-1**.) This last step—response—is essential, as it has been said that *surveillance without response is just documentation of misery.*

There are many different kinds of public health surveillance activities, ranging from periodic surveys to real-time reporting through direct communication from either

BOX 11-1 Biosurveillance Defined

In February 2010, the Centers for Disease Control and Prevention released a *National Biosurveillance Strategy for Human Health* V2.0. Within this strategy, CDC defined biosurveillance as follows:

Biosurveillance in the context of human health is a new term for the science and practice of managing health-related data and information for early warning of threats and hazards, early detection of events, and rapid characterization of the event so that effective actions can be taken to mitigate adverse health effects. It represents a new health information paradigm that seeks to integrate and efficiently manage health-related data and information across a range of information systems toward timely and accurate population health situation awareness.

The scope and function of biosurveillance includes the following:
- All hazards: including biological, chemical, radiological, nuclear, and explosives
- Defined by urgency and potential for multi-jurisdictional interest
- Urgent notifiable conditions and nonspecific and novel health events
- Ad hoc data gathering, analysis, and application of information
- Functions: Case Detection, Event Detection, Signal Validation, Event Characterization, Notification and Communication, and Quality Control and Improvement
- Supports rapid and efficient discharge of responsibilities for the International Health Regulations [IHR (2005)]

Source: U.S. Department of Health and Human Services, Centers for Disease Control and Prevention. *National Biosurveillance Strategy for Human Health.* February 2010. Available at: http://www.cdc.gov/osels/pdf/NBSHH_V2_FINAL.PDF. Accessed December 15, 2010.

laboratories or clinicians or warnings from advanced data algorithms designed to pick up unusual syndromes or behaviors. While surveys and surveillance of endemic diseases are essential to the public health community, it is the surveillance of emerging infections, unusual events, and potential public health emergencies that most inform public health preparedness and are the situations in which rapid detection is essential for saving lives. **Figure 11-2** shows the range of public health surveillance targets, arranged by priority (from national to international) and urgency of action.[4] While the

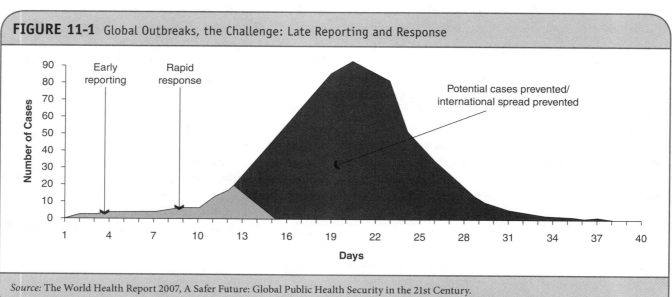

FIGURE 11-1 Global Outbreaks, the Challenge: Late Reporting and Response

Source: The World Health Report 2007, A Safer Future: Global Public Health Security in the 21st Century.

FIGURE 11-2 Public Health Surveillance Targets Arrayed by Urgency of Action and Priority

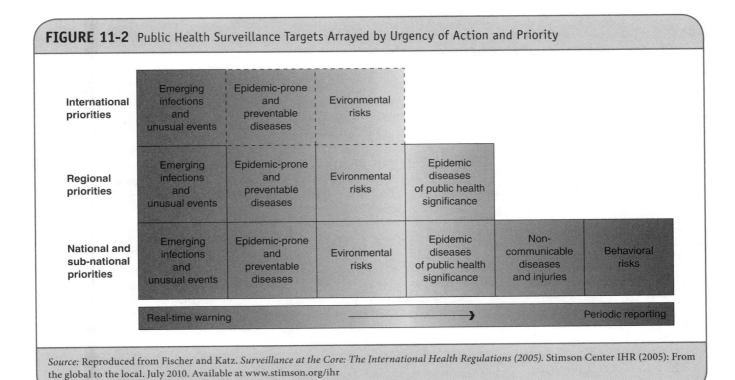

Source: Reproduced from Fischer and Katz. *Surveillance at the Core: The International Health Regulations (2005).* Stimson Center IHR (2005): From the global to the local. July 2010. Available at www.stimson.org/ihr

types of targets vary, effective surveillance for all requires adequate infrastructure, sufficient human capabilities, appropriate tools, and standardized processes.

Surveillance activities themselves involve multiple actors at different levels of government and private sectors. Detection of an unusual disease event almost always starts with an astute clinician who is able to discern that something is different/unusual/threatening about a particular patient or cluster of patients (be they human or animal), and who alerts authorities. Specimen samples must then be transferred in an appropriate manner to a laboratory with the proper equipment and expertise to perform accurate and reliable diagnostic tests. A communication network must be in place so that data from clinicians and laboratories feed into a system that allows for effective data analysis. In addition, hospitals may report into this system using discharge data or other markers. Pharmacists and other stores may report prescription and over-the-counter sales of drugs, as well as other indicator items, such as toilet paper sales. School or workplace absenteeism may be tracked to provide early indication of illness circulating in a community. All of these data may be actively collected by public health officials reaching out to all of the potential data sources or through passive surveillance, relying on the various actors to report events to authorities.

Regardless of how data are collected, all data must be integrated and analyzed to differentiate between expected levels of morbidity and mortality and indications of an unusual or unexpected event. The information collected should facilitate action so control measures can be taken. The data alone are not enough; trained public health professionals must analyze the data to determine proper actions.

POLICY DIRECTIVES

The importance of biosurveillance to public health preparedness and national and homeland security has been addressed in a variety of policy directives and legislation over the past decade. **Table 11-1**, produced by the Government Accountability Office (GAO), shows that there have been calls for an integrated, functional, domestic biosurveillance system starting with the Public Health Security and Bioterrorism Preparedness and Response Act of 2002. Further legislation in 2006 (Pandemic and All-Hazards Preparedness Act, PAHPA) and 2007 (Implementing Recommendations of the 9/11 Commission Act) reiterated the need for strong biosurveillance systems. PAHPA called for a near-real-time electronic system to enable detection, rapid response, and management of public health emergencies and other infectious disease outbreaks.[5](§ 202) The Implementing Recommendations of

TABLE 11-1 GAO Time Line of Laws and Presidential Directives Related to Biosurveillance

Date		
July 2002	Public Health Security and Bioterrorism Preparedness and Response Act of 2002	• Requires DHHS to establish an integrated system of public health alert communications and surveillance networks between and among federal, state, and local public health officials, and public and private health-related laboratories, hospitals, and other healthcare facilities.
January 2004	HSPD-9: Defense of United States Agriculture and Food	• Directs DOI, USDA, DHHS, and EPA to develop—for animals, plants, wildlife, food, human health, and water—robust, comprehensive, and fully coordinated surveillance and monitoring systems, including new tracking systems and integrated laboratory networks that use standardized protocols and procedures. • Directs DHS to create a biological threat awareness capacity to enhance detection and characterization of biological attacks that integrates and analyzes data on human, animal, and plant health; food; and water quality.
April 2004	HSPD-10: Biodefense for the 21st Century	• States that the federal government is working to develop an integrated and comprehensive system to rapidly recognize and characterize the dispersal of biological agents in human and animal populations, food, water, agriculture, and the environment to permit the recognition of a biological attack at the earliest possible moment and permit initiation of a robust response to prevent unnecessary loss of life, economic losses, and social disruption.
December 2006	Pandemic and All-Hazards Preparedness Act of 2006	• Requires DHHS to establish a near real-time electronic nationwide public health situational awareness capability through an interoperable network of systems to share data and information to enhance early detection of, rapid response to, and management of potentially catastrophic infectious disease outbreaks and other public health emergencies.
August 2007	Implementing Recommendations of the 9/11 Commission Act of 2007	• Requires DHS to establish a center to enhance the ability of the nation to rapidly identify, characterize, localize, and track a biological event of national concern by integrating and analyzing data relating to human health, animal, plant, food, and environmental monitoring systems.
October 2007	HSPD-21: Public Health and Medical Preparedness	• States that the United States must develop a nationwide, robust, and integrated biosurveillance capability, with connections to international disease surveillance systems, in order to provide timely warning and situational awareness.

Source: Reproduced from GAO Report: *Biosurveillance: Efforts to develop a national biosurveillance capability need a national strategy and a designated leader.* Available at http://www.gao.gov/new.items/d10645.pdf

the 9/11 Commission Act of 2007 called for a coordinated national biosurveillance capability, but the primary focus was on the role the Department of Homeland Security should play in providing an integrating center for all surveillance data.[6](§ 1101–1102)

The executive branch has released a series of policy directives and strategies highlighting the importance of disease surveillance and calling for a strong biosurveillance capability. In January 2004, the George W. Bush administration released HSPD 9, Defense of United States Agriculture and Food, which, among other things, directed a series of federal agen-

cies to develop a coordinated surveillance system, primarily for animals, plants, food, and water.[7] HSPD 10, Biodefense for the 21st Century, also released in 2004, reiterates the importance of early detection of a bioevent and the importance of an integrated surveillance system.[8] The major directive for surveillance released by the Bush administration, though, was HSPD 21, Public Health and Medical Preparedness, which explicitly calls for a robust, integrated, and comprehensive biosurveillance system as a primary pillar of public health preparedness (see **Box 11-2**).[1] HSPD 21 also focuses on the importance of connecting domestic biosurveillance to global disease surveillance systems to achieve effective early warning and characterization of disease outbreaks.[1]

The Obama administration, building on the recognition of the importance of strong biosurveillance for public health preparedness, released a series of strategies (all discussed in earlier chapters) that speak to the need for a robust, integrated surveillance system. The National Health Security Strategy of 2009 says, "A robust and integrated biosurveillance capability and effective leveraging of information in the private sector health care delivery system are especially important."[9] The National Strategy for Countering Biological Threats, also released in 2009, includes an entire section called "Building Global Capacity for Disease Surveillance, Detection, Diagnosis, and Reporting" in which the strategy commits the United States to working with partner countries and relevant international organizations to enable global surveillance networks to accurately report biothreat events in a manner that,

> Permits them to detect, identify, and report promptly any public, animal, or plant health or agricultural emergencies of international concern; Focuses on major population centers, known locations of endemic and epidemic disease and their vectors, and any known associated local terrorist or criminal threats; Is integrated and interoperable with their existing logistical infrastructure and sensitive to their public and agricultural health priorities; Is sustainable within the often limited resources of the country/region, either unilaterally or with other partners; Improves coordination between human, plant, and veterinary disease reporting systems, especially in relation to zoonotic diseases; and Is transparent and enables the sharing of information with international human, plant, and animal health agencies and the United States.[10]

Additionally, the National Security Strategy of 2010, the overarching strategy to address all security concerns of the United States, includes the following passage:

> Recognizing that the health of the world's population has never been more interdependent, we are improving our public health and medical capabilities on the front lines, including domestic and international disease surveillance, situational awareness, rapid and reliable development of medical countermeasures to respond to public health threats, preparedness education and training, and surge capacity of the domestic

BOX 11-2 HSPD 21: Public Health and Medical Preparedness Call for Robust Biosurveillance Capacity

The United States must develop a nationwide, robust, and integrated biosurveillance capability, with connections to international disease surveillance systems, in order to provide early warning and ongoing characterization of disease outbreaks in near real-time. Surveillance must use multiple modalities and an in-depth architecture. We must enhance clinician awareness and participation and strengthen laboratory diagnostic capabilities and capacity in order to recognize potential threats as early as possible. Integration of biosurveillance elements and other data (including human health, animal health, agricultural, meteorological, environmental, intelligence, and other data) will provide a comprehensive picture of the health of communities and the associated threat environment for incorporation into the national "common operating picture." A central element of biosurveillance must be an epidemiologic surveillance system to monitor human disease activity across populations. That system must be sufficiently enabled to identify specific disease incidence and prevalence in heterogeneous populations and environments and must possess sufficient flexibility to tailor analyses to new syndromes and emerging diseases. State and local government health officials, public and private sector health care institutions, and practicing clinicians must be involved in system design, and the overall system must be constructed with the principal objective of establishing or enhancing the capabilities of State and local government entities.

Source: The White House. *Homeland Security Presidential Directive 21: Public Health and Medical Preparedness.* October 18, 2007. Available at: http://www.fas.org/irp/offdocs/nspd/hspd-21.htm. Accessed November 5, 2010.

health care system to respond to an influx of patients due to a disaster or emergency. These capabilities include our ability to work with international partners to mitigate and contain disease when necessary.[11]

Taken together, the U.S. government has demonstrated an understanding of the importance of biosurveillance and has recognized the need for comprehensive, effective systems that can provide early detection, enable rapid response, and lead to efficient management of a public health emergency. The government also recognizes that more must be done to build a comprehensive and effective system. The next section of this chapter will describe the components of the domestic surveillance system and how they link to global efforts.

U.S. GOVERNMENT SURVEILLANCE PROGRAMS

Although the United States has numerous surveillance programs and systems at various levels of government and in the private sector to monitor disease, these programs and systems were developed separately for a variety of mission objectives, and as such are relatively uncoordinated.[12(p 2)]

While the government recognizes the importance of biosurveillance, and in practice the United States is probably one of the countries best suited to rapidly detect a public health event, the system that is currently in place is uncoordinated; relies on a multitude of separate data collection systems; and is challenged by the governmental infrastructure, which gives individual states the lead and authority for disease surveillance and only requires voluntary sharing of notifiable diseases with federal entities. Most of the resources and responsibilities for public health activities, including disease surveillance, lie at the local and state levels. Federal entities work with these state and local groups to encourage voluntary cooperation and information-sharing with the federal level.

There are numerous surveillance programs that are disease or syndrome specific, most of which are operated by CDC. In addition, there are a multitude of surveillance systems designed to capture data on disease events, including laboratory data. In 2010, the GAO described a selected set of such federally operated programs, which included more than 60 different programs, operated by the Department of Homeland Security, the Department of Defense, the Department of the Interior, the Environmental Protection Agency, the Department of Health and Human Services (including CDC and FDA), the Department of Agriculture, and the U.S. Postal Service.[13]

INTEGRATION EFFORTS

Given the enormity of the task and the multitude of surveillance systems that currently exist in the country, most experts and policy makers have recognized the need for a means to integrate data collection and analysis in a way that pools all of the available information, rapidly analyzes data, and provides early warning and response to public health emergen-cies. Several programs have tried to accomplish this, although to date, there are still challenges related to data and systems integration. The following sections discuss three of the bio-surveillance programs.

BioSense

BioSense was started by CDC in 2003 in response to the 2002 Bioterrorism Act; it was officially launched in 2004 and redesigned in 2007. The purpose of the program is to collect and analyze national near-real-time data from a variety of sources and, through the use of advanced algorithms, provide rapid assessments of disease trends. The program collects data on patient complaints from more than 550 acute care hospitals and 1,300 DoD and Veterans Affairs hospitals and clinics. It also collects sales data from more than 27,000 pharmacies. The data flow to the CDC BioIntelligence Center for analysis and are then shared back with the participating local and state entities. BioSense is currently trying to move away from collecting direct clinical data and, instead, emphasizing the collection of existing data from state and local entities to perform more of an integration service.[13(p 79),14]

National Biosurveillance Integration System

DHS hosts the National Biosurveillance Integration Center (NBIC). This center is designed to integrate and analyze data from human health, animal, plant, food, and environmental monitoring systems to create a single picture of bio-related activities. NBIC relies heavily on Argus, a federally funded but private surveillance system that filters media sources from around the world to collate disease-related information. The program also uses data from ESSENCE, a DoD surveillance program, as well as information from U.S. Fish and Wildlife Services and the EPA. While the NBIC concept is good, there have been significant challenges in implementing the program. Data from all federal agencies have not been readily shared and, when shared, are often in formats that need to be translated before integrated; analysis has not always been fully informed. The program is rebuilding and strengthening its capacity, and when fully operational and integrated with other agencies, it should be uniquely able to integrate data from a variety of sectors to gain a more complete picture of events.

Biowatch

Biowatch is an environmental monitoring program operated by the Department of Homeland Security, with partners at CDC and EPA. These are environmental "sniffers" designed to detect when a particular biological agent is present in the environment. These sniffers are currently located in approximately 30 cities. While earlier iterations of the monitors tended to lead to excessive false positives, later models are much more effective.[15]

GLOBAL SURVEILLANCE

> *The international community plays a key role in surveillance, detection, and communication of health security threats to their own nations, which may also pose a threat to our Nation.*[9(p 19)]

Because a biological threat can emerge anywhere, a weakness in the disease surveillance and response capacity in one part of the world is a potential risk to all nations. Therefore, it is vital that we take a global policy outlook in addition to national efforts so that we understand the global biosurveillance capacity, identify essential components of effective biosurveillance, and develop policies that will enable nations—particularly in resource poor environments—to establish systems that will quickly identify and respond to biological threats so that they may be contained prior to global spread.

The United States is committed to this concept through support of the World Health Organization's International Health Regulations [IHR (2005)] and the obligations under Article 44 of IHR (2005). Under Article 44 of the International Health Regulations (2005), States Parties are encouraged to provide technical and financial assistance to help other countries achieve their IHR core capacities, which are necessary to detect, respond to, and contain public health emergencies of international concern.[16(Art. 44)]

Multiple U.S. agencies are engaged in efforts to build disease surveillance capacity. The primary agencies supporting the broadest programs to promote disease surveillance and build epidemiologic and laboratory capacity around the world are the CDC, the Department of State (DOS), USAID, and DoD, which has dedicated the most resources to this endeavor.[17] (See **Table 11-2**.) Other agencies, including the intelligence community; the departments of Homeland Security, Commerce, Energy, and the Interior; EPA; and NASA have also been engaged in supporting global disease surveillance efforts. These combined efforts are designed to strengthen national capacities to detect, report, and respond to public health events, particularly public health emergencies. Some programs focus on developing workforce expertise, such as the CDC's Field Epidemiology Training Program (FETP and FELTP—for laboratory training). Some of the programs focus on infrastructure development and building laboratories for

TABLE 11-2 Major USG Global Surveillance Programs and Funding

Agency	Name of Program	FY2010 (Estimated)	FY2011 (Budget)
DHHS Centers for Disease Control and Prevention (CDC)	Global Disease Detection (GDD)	$37.7 million	$37.8 million
DHHS Centers for Disease Control and Prevention (CDC)	Early Warning Infectious Disease Surveillance System (EWIDS)	$5 million	$5 million
DoD Defense Threat Reduction Agency (DTRA)	Cooperative Biological Engagement Program (CBEP)	$133.3 million	$184.7 million
DoD Armed Forces Health Surveillance Center (AFHSC)	Global Emerging Infections Surveillance and Response System (GEIS)	$68.3 million	$55.0 million
DOS	Biosecurity Engagement Program (BEP)	$37 million	$37 million
USAID	Infectious Disease Surveillance, Emerging Pandemic Threats Program	$25 million	$25 million

Source: Data from Center for Biosecurity of UPMC. *International Disease Surveillance: United States Government Goals and Paths Forward.* Defense Technical Information Center. June 2010. Available at: http://www.dtic.mil/cgi-bin/GetTRDoc?AD=ADA528990&Location=U2&doc=GetTRDoc.pdf. Accessed December 15, 2010.

national and regional use. Several programs work on technological advances that can be utilized in both high- and low-resource environments to enable enhanced surveillance. And some of the programs provide support for pathogen discovery, outbreak investigation, and response and mitigation after the emergence of a public health event.

U.S. government–funded activities to promote disease surveillance capacity fit into a larger picture of global surveillance. A robust network of networks exists to support disease surveillance in all parts of the globe. These systems and networks overlap at the national, regional, and global levels and are designed to be coordinated at the international level by the WHO through the Global Outbreak Alert and Response Network (GOARN). The main electronic surveillance system utilized by the WHO to detect reports of disease through the media is the Global Public Health Information Network (GPHIN), a system developed by Health Canada. Other online information sources include less formal systems, such as PROMED, which is an online community of mostly health professionals sharing data about disease emergence. There are regional versions of this listserv as well, which also feed into the WHO. In addition to online sources, the WHO receives reports of disease emergence from ministries of health, WHO regional and national offices, laboratory networks, nongovernmental organizations (particularly those entities working on the ground in remote regions), militaries, and other entities within the United Nations system.[18]

Overall, there are a multitude of surveillance systems around the world—all designed to detect and report the emergence of a public health emergency as rapidly as possible to enable a timely response that will prevent morbidity and mortality. These systems range in effectiveness, and some parts of the world are better equipped than others in this arena. There appears, however, to be a strong commitment at the national and global policy levels to build stronger surveillance systems, and we should expect great strides in the next few years toward strengthening our domestic capabilities and building a comprehensive global system.

KEY WORDS

Surveillance
Biosurveillance
Situational awareness
HSPD 21
Biowatch
BioSense
National Biosurveillance Integration System
International Health Regulations
Global Outbreak Alert and Response Network

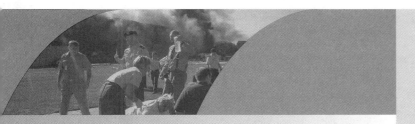

Discussion Questions

1. If you could design a biosurveillance system from scratch, what information would you want to collect and how? How would that information then be relayed to decision makers?

2. What are some of the successes and challenges of the current disease surveillance system in the United States?

3. Describe how countries' disease surveillance is interrelated. Who should be supporting global disease surveillance capacity building?

REFERENCES

1. The White House. *Homeland Security Presidential Directive 21: Public Health and Medical Preparedness.* Federation of American Scientists. October 18, 2007. Available at: http://www.fas.org/irp/offdocs/nspd/hspd-21.htm. Accessed November 5, 2010.

2. Raska K. National and International Surveillance of Communicable Diseases. *WHO Chronicle.* September 1966;20(9):315–321.

3. Thacker SB, Berkelman RL. Public Health Surveillance in the United States. *Epidemiologic Reviews.* 1988;10(1):164–190.

4. Fischer J, Katz R. *Surveillance at the Core: The International Health Regulations (2005).* Washington, DC: The Stimson Center, 2010.

5. Pandemic and All-Hazards Preparedness Act; Public Law No. 109-417.

6. Implementing Recommendations of the 9/11 Commission Act of 2007; Public Law No. 110-53.

7. The White House. *Homeland Security Presidential Directive 9: Defense of United States Agriculture and Food.* Federation of American Scientists. January 30, 2004. Available at: http://www.fas.org/irp/offdocs/nspd/hspd-9.html. Accessed November 5, 2010.

8. The White House. *Homeland Security Presidential Directive 10: Biodefense for the 21st Century.* Federation of American Scientists. April 28, 2004. Available at: http://www.fas.org/irp/offdocs/nspd/hspd-10.html. Accessed November 5, 2010.

9. U.S. Department of Health and Human Services. *National Health Security Strategy of The United States of America.* December 2009. Available at: http://www.phe.gov/Preparedness/planning/authority/nhss/strategy/Documents/nhss-final.pdf. Accessed July 25, 2010.

10. National Security Council. *National Strategy for Countering Biological Threats.* November 2009. Page 6. Available at: http://www.whitehouse.gov/sites/default/files/National_Strategy_for_Countering_BioThreats.pdf. Accessed September 10, 2010.

11. The White House. *National Security Strategy.* May 2010. Page 49. Available at: http://www.whitehouse.gov/sites/default/files/rss_viewer/national_security_strategy.pdf. Accessed July 25, 2010.

12. U.S. Government Accountability Office. *Biosurveillance: Developing a Collaboration Strategy Is Essential to Fostering Interagency Data and Resource Sharing.* December 2009. Available at: http://www.gao.gov/new.items/d10171.pdf. Accessed November 5, 2010.

13. U.S. Government Accountability Office. *Biosurveillance: Efforts to Develop a National Biosurveillance Capability Need a National Strategy and a Designated Leader.* June 2010. Available at: http://www.gao.gov/new.items/d10645.pdf. Accessed November 5, 2010.

14. Centers for Disease Control and Prevention. *BioSense.* September 14, 2009. Available at: http://www.cdc.gov/biosense/. Accessed November 5, 2010.

15. U.S. Department of Homeland Security. *Weapons of Mass Destruction and Biodefense Office.* August 13, 2009.

16. World Health Organization. *International Health Regulations (2005)* 2nd ed. 2008. Available at: http://whqlibdoc.who.int/publications/2008/9789241580410_eng.pdf.

17. Katz RL, López LM, Annelli JF, et al. U.S. Government Engagement in Support of Global Disease Surveillance. *BMC Public Health.* December 2010;10(Suppl 1). Available at: http://www.biomedcentral.com/content/pdf/1471-2458-10-S1-S13.pdf.

18. Grein TW, Kamara KBO, Rodier G, et al. Rumors of Disease in the Global Village: Outbreak Verification. *Emerging Infectious Diseases.* March–April 2000;6(2):97–102.

CHAPTER 12

Testing Preparedness: Natural Disasters and the Public Health Response

INTRODUCTION

Natural disasters occur all the time, in all regions of the world. Unlike a bioterrorism event, we know with absolute certainty that hurricanes will happen, earthquakes will occur near fault lines, active volcanoes will erupt, tornadoes will sweep through regions, snow will fall, fire will spread, and low-lying regions will flood. We know that every year, large populations will be stricken with influenza and occasionally a strain will emerge that can potentially lead to a pandemic. Public health emergency preparedness is as much about planning for and responding to these types of disasters as it is about responding to terrorist events. In fact, the public health community is much more likely to engage in disaster response to a naturally occurring event than to an intentional or accidental one. This chapter will examine how the public health community has responded to disasters and whether the response was appropriate and effective.

Public health professionals have long been engaged in disaster response. And as long as there have been emergencies, there have been medical personnel attending to the needs of populations. CDC started responding officially to disasters in the 1960s, when an Epidemic Intelligence Service (EIS) team traveled to Nigeria to help maintain public health programs in the middle of a civil war. Over the decades, CDC has developed public health and epidemiologic tools to address the realities of disaster situations and displaced populations. The public health community enters a disaster situation and establishes prevention and control measures, collects critical data to support response, and works to meet the short- and longer-term needs of the population.[1,2] Often, the most experienced public health and medical professionals on the ground during an emergency come from the nongovernmental organization (NGO) community, which has decades of experience responding to and helping populations recover from disasters. In fact, the American Red Cross, an NGO, has a federal charter to engage in disaster relief and has specific responsibilities outlined in the National Response Framework, based on its recognized expertise in this area.[3] In addition, military assets are utilized during emergencies to get qualified personnel to the event site quickly and, most important, to provide logistical support because some disasters require resources only the militaries of the world possess to reach isolated populations, bring supplies to remote regions, and establish care and living centers in harsh environments.[4,5]

Many disasters and public health emergencies draw out the best of humanity. People—in general—want to help. As a result, a wide assortment of organizations and individuals may respond to calls for assistance in the aftermath or in the midst of an event. Some of these organizations are well coordinated, systematic in their approach, and well versed in disaster response approaches. Others, particularly individual volunteers, have less formal training. In 1997, a group of NGOs, along with the International Federation of Red Cross and Red Crescent Societies, launched an initiative called the Sphere Project, which is designed to define and uphold guidelines for how the global community responds to disasters. Sphere produces a handbook, which illuminates core principles to govern humanitarian action, focusing on the rights of populations to protection and assistance. The project also works to promote a commitment to quality and accountability in the midst of humanitarian action.[6]

This chapter examines several major public health emergencies in the last few years, looks at the history of events, and describes the public health response. The chapter focuses on Hurricane Katrina and pandemic influenza. **Tables 12-1** and **12-2** illustrate the magnitude—measured in mortality—of

TABLE 12-1 Major Natural Disasters, 1900 to Present*

Date	Event	Location	Approximate Death Toll
January 12, 2010	Haiti Earthquake	Port-au-Prince, Haiti	230,000
December 26, 2004	Indian Ocean Tsunami	Indonesia, Thailand, Sri Lanka, India, and more	220,000 (+)
July 28, 1976	China Earthquake	Tangshan, China	242,000–655,000
November 13, 1970	Bhola Cyclone	Bangladesh	500,000
May–August 1931	Yellow River and Yangtze River floods	China	1–3.7 million
May 22, 1927	Xining Earthquake	Xining, China	200,000
September 1, 1923	Tokyo Earthquake and Fires	Tokyo, Japan	143,000
December 16, 1920	Haiyuan Earthquake	Haiyuan, China	200,000

*This is a select list of major natural disasters over the last 150 years.

Sources: Noji EK. *The Public Health Consequences of Disasters.* New York: Oxford University Press, 1997 (p 5); CBC News. *The World's Worst Natural Disasters: Calamities of the 20th and 21st Centuries.* August 30, 2010. Available at: http://www.cbc.ca/world/story/2008/05/08/f-natural-disasters-history. html?rdr=525. Accessed December 15, 2010; U.S. Agency for International Development, Office of U.S. Foreign Disaster Assistance. *Disaster History: Significant Data on Major Disasters Worldwide, 1900–Present.* August 1993. Available at: http://pdf.usaid.gov/pdf_docs/PNABP986.pdf. Accessed December 15, 2010; Associated Press. Haiti Raises Earthquake Toll to 230,000. *The Washington Post.* February 10, 2010. Available at: http://www.washingtonpost.com/ wp-dyn/content/article/2010/02/09/AR2010020904447.html. Accessed December 15, 2010; U.S. Agency for International Development. *USAID Disaster Assistance, Indian Ocean Tsunami.* May 30, 2007. Available at: http://www.usaid.gov/our_work/humanitarian_assistance/disaster_assistance/countries/ indian_ocean/template/index.html. Accessed December 15, 2010.

TABLE 12-2 Influenza Pandemic, 1900–Present

Year	Name	Strain	Approximate death toll worldwide
1918	Spanish flu	H1N1	50 million worldwide
1957	Asian Influenza	H2N2	2 million
1968	Hong Kong Influenza	H3N2	1 million
2003–2005	Avian Influenza*	H5N1	500
2009	Swine flu, or H1N1	H1N1	18,000

*Avian Influenza was not a pandemic, in that there was no sustained human-to-human transmission or large-scale spread to multiple regions of the world, but the strain had "pandemic potential" and resulted in intense international attention.

Sources: Ebrahim GJ. Avian Flu and Influenza Pandemics in Human Populations. *Journal of Tropical Pediatrics.* 2004;50(4):192–194; Trust for America's Health. *Pandemic Flu and the Potential for U.S. Economic Recession: A State-by-State Analysis.* March 2007. Available at: http://healthyamericans.org/reports/ flurecession/FluRecession.pdf. Accessed December 15, 2010; Kilbourne ED. Influenza Pandemics of the 20th Century. *Emerging Infectious Diseases.* January 2006;12(1):9–14; Taubenberger JK, Morens DM. 1918 Influenza: The Mother of All Pandemics. *Emerging Infectious Diseases.* January 2006;12(1):15–22; World Health Organization. Cumulative Number of Confirmed Human Cases of Avian Influenza A/(H5N1) Reported to WHO. Global Alert and Response (GAR). August 31, 2010. Available at: http://www.who.int/csr/disease/avian_influenza/country/cases_table_2010_08_31/en/index.html. Accessed December 15, 2010.

major natural disasters and pandemics, and **Box 12-1** (Indian Ocean Tsunami) and **Box 12-2** (Haiti Earthquake) provide information about other major natural disasters in recent history.

BOX 12-1 Indian Ocean Tsunami

On December 26, 2004, an earthquake with a magnitude between 9.1 and 9.3 struck off the northwest coast of Sumatra, Indonesia. The undersea earthquake sparked a tsunami that traveled throughout the Indian Ocean, affecting 12 countries in south Asia, Southeast Asia, and East Africa. (See **Figure 12-1.**) The hardest hit countries were Indonesia, Sri Lanka, India, and Thailand, and overall more than 220,000 were killed and a million individuals left without a home. Basic infrastructure was destroyed, entire communities were swept to sea, and social services—including health care—in affected regions were wiped out.

The international community, led by WHO and UNICEF, coordinated numerous NGOs, governmental aid, and military assistance to provide disaster relief and humanitarian assistance to the affected regions. In addition to traditional public health and medical response needs, such as rapid restoration of safe drinking water, this particular response required strong military logistical support to reach remote regions with destroyed infrastructure. In addition, aid agencies had to be particularly attentive to the problem of child trafficking and ensure that children orphaned by the tsunami or separated from their families during the disaster were protected from trafficking.

Sources: Margesson R. *CRS Report for Congress: Indian Ocean Earthquake and Tsunami: Humanitarian Assistance and Relief Operations.* Federation of American Scientists. February 10, 2005. Available at: http://www.fas.org/sgp/crs/row/RL32715.pdf. Accessed November 5, 2010; and Dannheisser R. *Aid Efforts Continue Well After Devastating 2004 Tsunami.* America.gov. October 29, 2007. Available at: http://www.america.gov/st/washfile-english/2007/October/20071029081347AKllennoCcM0.4600946.html. Accessed November 5, 2010.

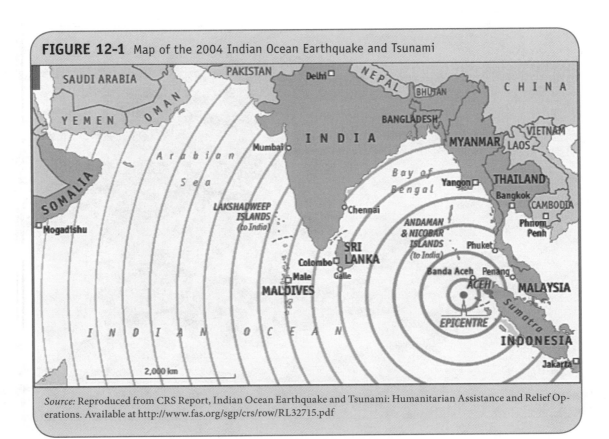

FIGURE 12-1 Map of the 2004 Indian Ocean Earthquake and Tsunami

Source: Reproduced from CRS Report, Indian Ocean Earthquake and Tsunami: Humanitarian Assistance and Relief Operations. Available at http://www.fas.org/sgp/crs/row/RL32715.pdf

BOX 12-2 Haiti Earthquake

On January 12, 2010, a 7.0 magnitude earthquake struck 10 miles from the Haitian capital of Port-au-Prince. (See **Figure 12-2.**) Almost 3 million people required emergency assistance, and more than 230,000 died. The quake destroyed the already fragile health care infrastructure. CDC defined the public health priorities as those for any natural disaster—reduce and prevent further deaths, illness, and injuries; determine and meet critical needs for water, sanitation, health care, and food; verify status of health care facilities and assist in setting up health care services; assess emergency health needs, including those of mothers and infants; provide health education; and conduct disease surveillance. Faculty and students from schools of public health across the United States engaged in disaster response and relief efforts to manage displacement camps, coordinate refugees, assist with hospital surge efforts, conduct public health assessments, and coordinate supplies. These public health professionals joined clinical volunteers from hospitals and schools of medicine and nursing to provide both emergency and ongoing health care.

   The Haiti case demonstrates the importance of overall governance to a successful response effort. In October 2010, with most of the displaced persons still living in tent cities and poor access to clean water, a cholera epidemic erupted; at the time of this writing, the epidemic has affected more than 104,000 people and claimed more than 2,300 lives.

Sources: Centers for Disease Control and Prevention. *Public Health Issues and Priorities for the Haiti Earthquake.* January 14, 2010. Available at: http://www.bt.cdc.gov/disasters/earthquakes/healthconcerns_haiti.asp. Accessed November 5, 2010; Association of Schools of Public Health. *Haitian Earthquake Relief: Schools of Public Health Respond.* Available at: http://www.asph.org/document.cfm?page=1141. Accessed November 5, 2010; and Fox News Latino. More Than 2,300 Now Dead from Cholera in Haiti. *Fox News Latino.* December 14, 2010. Available at: http://latino.foxnews.com/latino/health/2010/12/14/dead-cholera-haiti/. Accessed December 15, 2010; World Health Organization, Pan American Health Organization. *PAHO Responds to Cholera Outbreak in Haiti.* November 3, 2010. Available at: http://new.paho.org/disasters/index.php?option=com_content&task=view&id=1423&Itemid=1. Accessed November 5, 2010.

FIGURE 12-2 Haiti Earthquake Radius

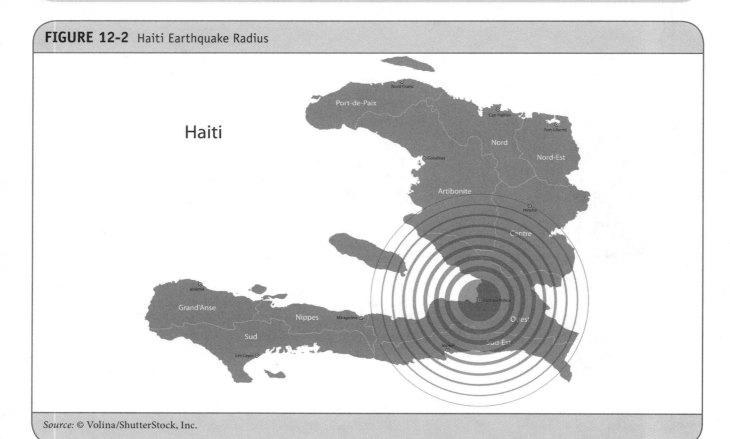

Source: © Volina/ShutterStock, Inc.

HURRICANE KATRINA

On August 29, 2005, Hurricane Katrina landed on the Gulf Coast of the United States, reaching Mississippi, Louisiana, and Alabama. (See **Figure 12-3** for map of where Katrina came ashore.) It came ashore with 115 to 130 mph winds, and brought with it a storm surge as high as 27 feet of water that went between 6 and 12 miles inland and flooded about 80% of the city of New Orleans. Approximately 93,000 square miles were affected, resulting in 1,300 fatalities, 2 million displaced persons, 300,000 homes destroyed, and almost $100 billion in property damage.[7(pp 5–9)]

Katrina was the worst domestic natural disaster in recent history, but the consequences of the event were heightened by a faltering levee system designed by the U.S. Army Corps of Engineers and a failure of government at all levels to properly prepare for and respond to the disaster. (**Figure 12-4** depicts the impact of Katrina in comparison to past hurricanes in the

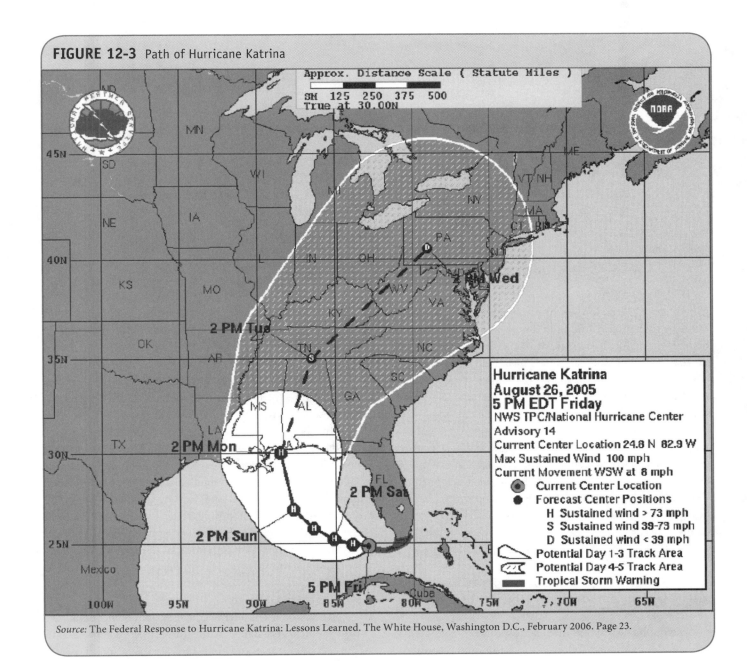

FIGURE 12-3 Path of Hurricane Katrina

Source: The Federal Response to Hurricane Katrina: Lessons Learned. The White House, Washington D.C., February 2006. Page 23.

FIGURE 12-4 U.S. Natural Disasters That Caused the Most Death and Damage to Property in Each Decade 1900–2005. Damage in Third Quarter 2005 Dollars. Major 2004 Hurricanes Combined and Analyzed Together

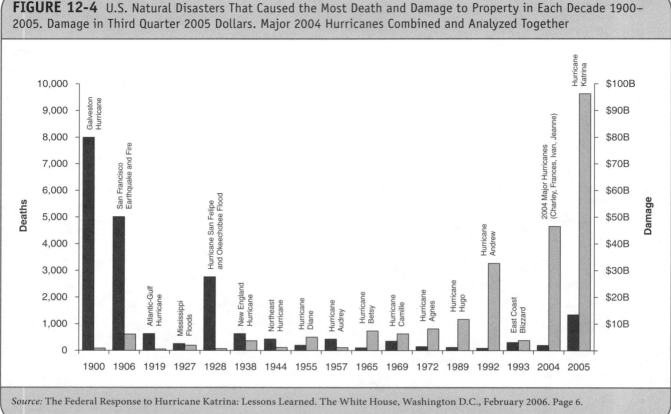

Source: The Federal Response to Hurricane Katrina: Lessons Learned. The White House, Washington D.C., February 2006. Page 6.

United States.) First, long-term warnings went unheeded. It was clear that a hurricane of this type would eventually hit the region, and local and state officials—even after running exercises based on such a scenario—failed to properly prepare. Local and state officials were unable to evacuate all of the citizens; struggled with logistics; and did not make proper preparations for dealing with vulnerable populations, including nursing home residents. The federal government failed to adequately anticipate the needs of the state and local authorities, and the insufficient coordination resulted in not enough resources getting to the right populations at the right time.

In 2005, the National Response Plan and the National Incident Management System existed (see previous chapters), but the experience with Katrina made it clear that they were not well understood or even widely read.[7,8,9] Multiple levels of government did not have a common operating picture, there was limited communication, and there were misunderstandings about who was in charge of which aspects of the response.

The public health and medical response coordinated by the federal government followed the traditional response to a flood or hurricane: focus on sanitation and hygiene, water safety, surveillance and infection control, environmental health, and access to care.[9,10] Katrina, though, also presented unique challenges, such as the inability of displaced persons to manage chronic disease conditions and access medications, death and illness from dehydration, and mental health concerns associated with the widespread devastation.

Almost all offices and branches of DHHS became involved in the federal response to Katrina. The CDC sent staff to the affected areas, deployed the Strategic National Stockpile (SNS) to provide drugs and medical supplies, and developed public health and occupational health guidance. FDA issued recommendations for handling drugs that might have been affected by the flood. NIH set up a phone-based medical consultation service for providers in the region. The Substance Abuse and Mental Health Services Administration (SAMHSA) set up crisis counseling assistance and provided emergency response grants.[9]

The National Disaster Medical System deployed 50 Disaster Medical Assistance Teams (described in **Box 12-3**) to try to accommodate and treat hurricane victims. Disaster

BOX 12-3 Disaster Medical Assistance Teams

Disaster Medical Assistance Teams (DMATs) are part of the National Disaster Medical System operated by DHHS and are composed of medical personnel, including physicians, nurses, paramedics, and other health professionals. Team members may be volunteers from the private sector or federal employees, who train together and can be called up to respond to emergencies—at which point all team members are activated as intermittent federal employees. Teams are usually activated for a 2-week period. The teams are designed to be rapid-response units to supplement local medical care during an emergency. They triage, provide care, and help—when necessary—evacuate patients.

Source: U.S. Department of Health and Human Services. Assistant Secretary for Preparedness Response. *Disaster Medical Assistance Team (DMAT).* October 21, 2010. Available at: http://www.phe.gov/Preparedness/responders/ndms/teams/Pages/dmat.aspx. Accessed December 15, 2010.

Mortuary Operational Response Teams also deployed to help process bodies. The DoD set up field hospitals at the New Orleans International Airport and aboard naval vessels. The Department of Veterans Affairs evacuated both of its local hospitals—one prior to the storm, one afterwards.[9]

Even with all of this activity, serious challenges existed for the public health and medical response. Not all hospitals and nursing homes were evacuated in advance of the storm. Once patients were evacuated, medical care was uncoordinated and underresourced and care had to be triaged. Patients were moved without their loved ones and separated from medical records.

In the aftermath of Katrina, the White House released a "lessons learned" report, with 17 lessons and 125 recommendations for strengthening disaster response. Included in these recommendations was the need to revise the National Response Plan and specifically strengthen capability and command and control of assets associated with ESF 8 (Public Health and Medical Response—Emergency Support Function). These changes were included in the revised National Response Framework. Also, in the wake of Katrina, the government has expanded the role of the assistant secretary for Preparedness and Response at DHHS and is better coordinating and training rapidly deployable public health and medical teams.[7]

AVIAN AND PANDEMIC INFLUENZA

From 2003 to 2005, avian influenza circulated throughout Southeast Asia and along the flyways of migratory birds. Wild birds carried the H5N1 virus and passed it to domestic birds. Poultry became sick and, in some cases, passed the virus to humans in close contact with the birds. (See **Figure 12-5** for map of flyways and poultry density in Southeast Asia.) Global health experts watched the virus with great trepidation because the case fatality rate for reported cases in humans was extremely high (more than 50%) and the world feared that H5N1 would cause the next pandemic. As it turned out, there were only sparse cases of human-to-human transmission, and to date, no sustained human-to-human transmission necessary for a pandemic, but the virus continues to circulate.[11,12]

In response to H5N1 and predictions that if it became a pandemic it would have a devastating toll on human life, economies, and stability, a global effort was made to engage in pandemic preparedness. The WHO created pandemic plans.[13] Every country, following WHO guidance, created national pandemic plans. In the United States, the White House released a pandemic plan, DHHS released its own pandemic plan, and each state was responsible for designing its own pandemic plans.[14] **Box 12-4** presents a list of some of the plans developed by federal agencies.

The United States established what is now known as the North American Leaders Summit partnership with Canada and Mexico, and one aspect of the partnership was the development of a trilateral avian and pandemic plan to ensure communication and coordination during a pandemic response.[15] The Defense Department was directed to use funds from a congressional supplement for avian and pandemic influenza surveillance to increase surveillance, laboratory support, and communication.[16] U.S. government agencies aided in surveillance efforts around the globe, particularly in regions along the wildlife flyways.

During this time, the International Health Regulations (2005) were approved by the World Health Assembly, and in 2006, one year before they officially entered into force, the

FIGURE 12-5 Avian Influenza Flyways and Poultry Density

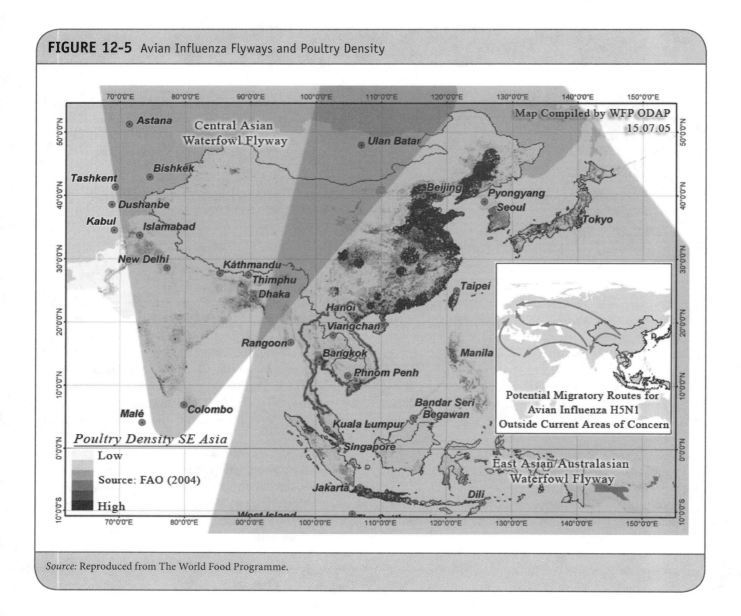

Source: Reproduced from The World Food Programme.

World Health Assembly agreed to comply voluntarily with the provisions of the IHR as they pertain to avian and pandemic influenza.[17]

H1N1

In April 2009, novel influenza A (H1N1) emerged in North America. Less than 2 months later, the virus was officially declared a pandemic by the World Health Organization, and it was declared the first public health emergency of international concern (PHEIC) under the International Health Regulations (2005). By the end of the pandemic in August 2010, the virus had spread to every country, although fortunately, the mortality rate remained low.

The preparedness activities for H5N1 allowed the public health community to mount an aggressive and coordinated response to H1N1, although it also highlighted areas for improvement. Because the pandemic did not turn out to be severe, it served as a "dry run" for how the public health community would respond to a larger-scale event. As Trust for America's Health wrote, "Overall, the H1N1 outbreak has shown that the investment the country has made in preparing for a potential pandemic flu has significantly improved U.S. capabilities for a large scale infectious disease outbreak, but it has also revealed how quickly the nation's core public health capacity would be overwhelmed if the outbreak were more widespread and more severe."[18(p 1)]

BOX 12-4　Pandemic Preparedness Plans: Select Plans and Strategies (Available at flu.gov)

On flu.gov, the federal pandemic flu website, the government lists all of the federal-level strategies and plans available on pandemic preparedness. Here is a selection of entries from that website:

- *The National Strategy for Pandemic Influenza* (White House)
- *The Implementation Plan for the National Strategy* (White House)
- *Vaccine Prioritization* (U.S. Department of Health and Human Services; U.S. Department of Homeland Security)
- *Department of Defense Implementation Plan for Pandemic Influenza* (U.S. Department of Defense)
- *HHS Pandemic Influenza Implementation Plan—Part 1* (U.S. Department of Health and Human Services)
  - *Pandemic Planning Updates from 2006–2009*
- *VA Pandemic Influenza Plan* (U.S. Department of Veterans Affairs)
- *Pandemic Planning Report* (U.S. Department of Agriculture)
- *Avian Influenza (Bird Flu)* (U.S. Department of Agriculture)
- *Avian Flu* (U.S. Environmental Protection Agency)
- *Avian Influenza* (U.S. Geological Survey, National Wildlife Health Center)
- *Guidance on Preparing Workplaces for an Influenza Pandemic* (Occupational Safety and Health Administration)
- *Emergency Planning: Influenza Outbreak* (U.S. Department of Education)
- *Pandemic Influenza Preparedness, Response, and Recovery Guide for Critical Infrastructure and Key Resources* (U.S. Department of Homeland Security)
- *Pandemic Flu Planning Resources* (U.S. Fire Administration; U.S. Department of Homeland Security)
- *National Avian Influenza Surveillance Information* (U.S. Geological Survey)
- *EMS Pandemic Influenza Guidelines for Statewide Adoption* (National Highway Traffic Safety Administration)
- *Recommendations for Protocol Development for 9-1-1 Personnel* (National Highway Traffic Safety Administration)

It was the Department of Defense influenza surveillance system established with congressional authorization to fight avian influenza that picked up the first two cases of H1N1 in the United States. The Revised International Health Regulations worked as designed for notification to the WHO of a potential public health emergency of international concern. The North American Leaders Summit agreement among Canada, the United States, and Mexico allowed for seamless sharing of information. A PHEIC was declared by the rules of the IHR, and a pandemic was declared by the rules of the WHO pandemic plan. (Note: While the pandemic followed the WHO guidelines, there was pushback that the guidelines themselves did not take severity of the virus into account.) Nations utilized their pandemic plans to the extent they were flexible enough to account for a virus like H1N1 emerging in North America. Most nations followed evidence-based guidance, although some—operating within their own sovereign right—disregarded WHO recommendations and enacted their own policies, sometimes at the expense of travel, trade, and individual rights.[19,20]

The Strategic National Stockpile was used to dispense H1N1 vaccines to the states. The states were then responsible for distribution of the vaccine, as outlined in domestic planning documents. Public health officials communicated with the public, sharing data as they became available. With all of this, however, there was still a lot to be learned regarding preparedness and response activities.

While pandemic plans were in place, local and state health departments did not have sufficient resources to carry out the plans—highlighting the importance of a consistent public health workforce. Also, because the virus was not the H5N1 scenario used for the creation of the pandemic plans, planners realized the importance of producing adaptable and flexible plans. Another issue of concern was the closing of schools and social gatherings to reduce transmission. While school closings had long been a part of pandemic planning, public health officials were unprepared for the disruption such closings caused, and asking people to stay home when sick in the absence of paid sick leave was problematic and will most likely require a legislative solution.

Some recommendations for future action developed by the Trust for America's Health and the Center for Biosecurity of UPMC include the following:

- Maintaining the Strategic National Stockpile.
- Developing more thorough strategies for school closings, sick leave, and community mitigations.
- Improving vaccine development and production capabilities.
- Ensuring a robust local and state health workforce.
- Planning for surge capacity.
- Developing regulations and plans to care for the uninsured and underinsured.[18]

The public health community needs to better manage expectations within communities and use faster surveillance to get better information to the public sooner.[21]

Overall, the public health community continues to learn from each emergency and plan for the next. While no plan is perfect, all of the efforts toward preparedness over the past decade have helped the public health community ready itself for emergencies. With each event, we learn more. We also learn that a large-scale event will no doubt overwhelm the medical infrastructure and tax all of our planning efforts, so we must do as much as possible to prepare for such situations.

KEY WORDS

Natural disasters
Avian influenza
Pandemic
Hurricane Katrina
Tsunami
Earthquake
H1N1

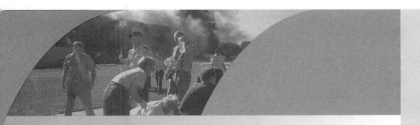

Discussion Questions

1. What are other natural disasters that have occurred, and how did the public health community respond?

2. Characterize the response to Hurricane Katrina. What do you believe are the most important lessons to be learned for future events?

3. Review the pandemic plans put in place in response to H5N1. Where do you think these plans succeeded? Identify some of the potential problems with the plans.

4. How could the United States and the world have better responded to the H1N1 pandemic?

REFERENCES

1. Noji EK. *The Public Health Consequences of Disasters*. New York: Oxford University Press, 1997.

2. Gregg MB, ed. *The Public Health Consequences of Disasters. CDC Monograph*. Atlanta, GA: Centers for Disease Control and Prevention, 1989.

3. The American National Red Cross. *The Federal Charter of the American Red Cross*. Available at: http://www.redcross.org/portal/site/en/menuitem.d229a5f06620c6052b1ecfbf43181aa0/?vgnextoid=39c2a8f21931f110VgnVCM10000089f0870aRCRD&cpsextcurrchannel=1. Accessed December 15, 2010.

4. Wiharta S, Ahmad H, Haine JY, Löfgren J, Randall T. *The Effectiveness of Foreign Military Assets in Natural Disaster Response*. Stockholm International Peace Research Institute, 2008.

5. VanRooyen M, Leaning J. After the Tsunami—Facing the Public Health Challenges. *The New England Journal of Medicine*. February 2005;352(5):435–438.

6. About Us. *The Sphere Project*. Available at: http://www.sphereproject.org/content/view/91/58/lang,english/. Accessed November 5, 2010.

7. The White House. *The Federal Response to Hurricane Katrina Lessons Learned*. February 2006. Available at: http://library.stmarytx.edu/acadlib/edocs/katrinawh.pdf. Accessed September 10, 2010.

8. U.S. Senate Committee on Homeland Security and Governmental Affairs. *Hurricane Katrina: A Nation Still Unprepared (Senate Report 109-322)*. Washington, DC: U.S. Government Printing Office, 2006.

9. Lister SA. CRS Report for Congress: *Hurricane Katrina: The Public Health and Medical Response*. U.S. Department of State, Foreign Press Centers. September 21, 2005. Available at: http://fpc.state.gov/documents/organization/54255.pdf. Accessed November 5, 2010.

10. Greenough PG, Kirsch TD. Public Health Response—Assessing Needs. *The New England Journal of Medicine*. October 2005;353(15):1544–1546.

11. World Health Organization, Western Pacific Region. *Avian Influenza*. Available at: http://www.wpro.who.int/health_topics/avian_influenza/. Accessed November 5, 2010.

12. World Health Organization, Western Pacific Region. *Avian Influenza Still a Threat, Says WHO*. March 24, 2010. Available at: http://www.wpro.who.int/media_centre/press_releases/pr_20100324.htm. Accessed November 5, 2010.

13. Flu.gov. *Global Activities*. Available at: http://flu.gov/professional/global/index.html. Accessed November 5, 2010.

14. Flu.gov. *State Pandemic Plans*. Available at: http://flu.gov/professional/states/stateplans.html. Accessed November 5, 2010.

15. Security and Prosperity Partnership of North America. *North American Plan for Avian & Pandemic Influenza*. August 2007. Available at: http://www.spp-psp.gc.ca/eic/site/spp-psp.nsf/vwapj/pandemic-influenza.pdf/$FILE/pandemic-influenza.pdf. Accessed November 5, 2010.

16. Armed Forces Health Surveillance Center. *Global Emerging Infections Surveillance and Response System (GEIS) Operations*. Available at: http://www.afhsc.mil/geisPartners. Accessed November 5, 2010.

17. World Health Organization. The World Health Assembly Adopts Resolution WHA59.2 on Application of the International Health Regulations (2005) to Strengthen Pandemic Preparedness and Response. Available at: http://www.who.int/ihr/wharesolution2006/en/index.html. Accessed November 5, 2010.

18. Trust for America's Health. *Pandemic Flu Preparedness: Lessons from the Frontlines*. June 2009. Available at: http://healthyamericans.org/assets/files/pandemic-flu-lesson.pdf. Accessed November 5, 2010.

19. Katz R. Use of Revised International Health Regulations during Influenza A (H1N1) Epidemic, 2009. *Emerging Infectious Diseases*. August 2009;15(8):1165–1170.

20. Katz R, Fischer J. The Revised International Health Regulations: A Framework for Global Pandemic Response. *Global Health Governance Journal*. Spring 2010;3(2). Available at: http://ghgj.org/Katz%20and%20Fischer_The%20Revised%20International%20Health%20Regulations.pdf.

21. Watson M. The 2009 H1N1 Experience: Policy Implications for Future Infectious Disease Emergencies—Conference Brief. *UPMC Center for Biosecurity*. Available at: http://www.upmc-biosecurity.org/website/events/2010_h1n1/pdf/2010-03-05-H1N1-Conference_Brief.pdf. Accessed November 5, 2010.

CHAPTER 13

From Local Preparedness to Global Governance of Disease: The Path to Security

LEARNING OBJECTIVES

By the end of this chapter, the reader will be able to:

- Identify local and state activities that contribute to public health preparedness.
- Analyze legal guidelines for preparedness.
- Examine the role of quarantine and isolation in public health preparedness and how these steps may be taken.
- Describe how local efforts link with global activities to promote health security.

INTRODUCTION

Most of this book has focused on the role of the U.S. federal government in establishing infrastructure, policy, and guidance for improving public health preparedness and addressing the threats posed to population health. While a strong federal policy and infrastructure is essential, public health professionals recognize that most public health activities occur at the local and state levels. Clinical care is an essential component of public health, yet that care is not conducted in Washington, DC. It is in every doctor's office, hospital, and clinic around the country. Disease surveillance is essential, but it starts with detection of an unusual event by an astute clinician and a capable laboratory, wherever the event emerges. Not only is this a reality in practice, it is codified by the Tenth Amendment of the Constitution: "The powers not delegated to the United States by the Constitution, nor prohibited by it to the States, are reserved to the States respectively, or to the people." This means that police powers, including the powers to regulate health and safety, are the responsibility of the states. The federal government can and must support public health

preparedness domestically because it must build relations globally to ensure an effective worldwide system for preparedness, information sharing, and collaboration in preventing, detecting, reporting, and responding to public health threats. It is the state and local entities, however, that are relied on to implement policies, build infrastructure, and interface with local populations to promote health security. This is the case in the United States, as it is throughout the world.

In this chapter, we will look at state and local efforts to build public health preparedness. There have been major successes over the past decade, yet significant challenges remain. This chapter also examines the differentiation among state, local, and federal authorities for containing an infectious disease, with specific emphasis on quarantine regulations.

Finally, we will discuss how these local and state activities line up with global efforts to strengthen public health preparedness.

LOCAL AND STATE PREPAREDNESS ACTIVITIES

Public health professionals, supported by their professional associations—including the American Public Health Association (APHA), the Council of State and Territorial Epidemiologists (CSTE), the Association of Public Health Laboratories (APHL), the Association of State and Territorial Health Officers (ASTHO), and the National Association of County and City Health Officials (NACCHO)—and funded primarily by the CDC and DHHS/ASPR have been building preparedness capacity in several key areas. These functional areas include laboratory and epidemiologic capacity, communication, hospital preparedness, community resilience, and response capability.

FIGURE 13-1 U.S. Population within 100 Miles of a Laboratory in the Laboratory Response Network (LRN)

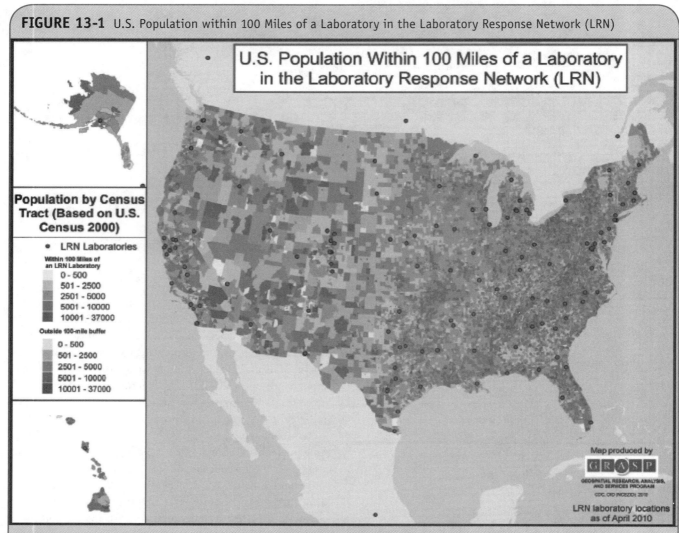

Source: Reproduced from U.S. Centers for Disease Control and Prevention. *Public Health Preparedness: Strengthening the Nation's Emergency Response State by State.* Centers for Disease Control and Prevention, Office of Public Health Preparedness and Response. September 2010. U.S. Centers for Disease Control and Prevention. Available at: http://www.bt.cdc.gov/publications/2010phprep/pdf/complete_PHPREP_report.pdf

Laboratory and Epidemiologic Capacity

The CDC has funded public health laboratories in every state and Washington, DC, as part of a cooperative agreement for preparedness. These laboratories are part of what is known as the Laboratory Response Network (LRN), which is a network of local, state, federal, and global labs with the capability to test for biological and chemical agents. As of 2008, there were 151 LRN laboratories throughout the United States that could test for agents.[1] Most of these laboratories can be reached at all times and rapidly identify certain bacteria. **Figure 13-1** shows the national distribution of LRN laboratories in relation to population. **Table 13-1** is from a CDC report released in September 2010 describing the state of laboratory capabilities in regard to public health preparedness and identification of biological and chemical agents. Overall, the laboratories are performing well but could be more efficient and effective, especially with additional funding and a more consistent workforce.

Every locality requires competent epidemiological capacity to support surveillance to detect public health threats. Epidemiologists are crucial to this endeavor because they are the ones on the front lines investigating public health events,

TABLE 13-1 National Snapshot of Laboratory Activities

Laboratories: General

Maintaining core laboratory functions during an emergency	Status of laboratory continuity of operations plan (COOP) for 50 states and DC: • **23 out of 51** had a state public health laboratory COOP • **15 out of 51** had a state COOP that included laboratory operations • **13 out of 51** had a COOP that was under development *APHL; 8/31/2007–8/30/2008*
Ensuring availability of Laboratory Response Network (LRN) laboratory results for decision making	**53 out of 54** states and localities had a standardized electronic data system capable of messaging laboratory results between LRN laboratories and also to CDC *CDC, OSELS; as of 9/30/2008*

Laboratories: Biological Capabilities

Participation in LRN for biological agents	**148 out of 151** LRN laboratories were reference laboratories that could test for biological agents The remaining 3 LRN laboratories were national laboratories that could test for biological agents *CDC, OID (NCEZID); as of 9/30/2008*
Assessing if laboratory emergency contacts could be reached 24/7	**135 out of 151** LRN laboratories were successfully contacted during a non-business hours telephone drill *CDC, OID (NCEZID); 8/2008*
Evaluating LRN laboratory capabilities	**261 out of 277** proficiency tests were passed by LRN reference and/or national laboratories *CDC, OID (NCEZID); 1/2008–9/2008*
Rapid identification of disease-causing bacteria by PulseNet laboratories	Rapidly identified *E. coli O 157:H7* using advanced DNA tests (PFGE): • **50 out of 50** states performed tests on *E. coli O157:H7* samples • **29 out of 50** of the states that performed tests submitted at least 90% of test results to the PulseNet database within 4 working days *CDC, OPHPR (DSLR); 8/31/2007–8/9/2008* Rapidly identified L. monocytogenes using advanced DNA tests (PFGF): • **32 out of 50** states performed tests on L. monocytogenes samples • **18 out of 32** of the states that performed tests submitted at least 90% of test results to the PulseNet database within 4 working days *CDC, OPHPR (DSLR); 8/31/2007–8/9/2008*
Assessing laboratory competency and reporting through exercises	**49 out of 51** public health laboratories in 50 states and DC conducted exercises to assess the competency of sentinel laboratories to rule out bioterrorism agents *APHL; 8/31/2007–8/30/2008* Ability of CDC–funded LRN laboratories* to contact the CDC Emergency Operations Center within 2 hours during LRN notification drill: • **35 out of 54** laboratories passed • **15 out of 54** laboratories did not participate • **4 out of 54** laboratories did not pass *There is one CDC-funded LRN laboratory in DC and in each state, with the exception of CA, IL, and NY, which each have two. *CDC, OID (NCEZID); 3/2008*

Laboratories: Chemical Capabilities

Participation in LRN for chemical agents (LRN-C)	56 LRN-C laboratories in states and localities could respond if the public was exposed to chemical agents: • **10 out of 56** are Level 1 laboratories (most advanced testing capabilities) • **37 out of 56** are Level 2 laboratories (testing capabilities for limited panel of agents) • **9 out of 56** are Level 3 laboratories (specimen collection, storage, and shipment) *CDC, ONDIEH (NCEH); as of 9/14/2009*

(continued)

TABLE 13-1 National Snapshot of Laboratory Activities *(Continued)*

Evaluating LRN-C laboratory capabilities through proficiency testing	**34 out of 47** Level 1 and/or Level 2 LRN-C laboratories successfully demonstrated all six core methods to rapidly detect chemical agents **26 out of 47** Level 1 and/or Level 2 LRN-C laboratories successfully demonstrated at least one additional method to rapidly detect chemical agents *CDC, ONDIEH (NCEH); as of 9/14/2009*
Assessing LRN-C laboratory capabilities through exercises	LRN-C laboratories' ability to collect, package, and ship samples properly during LRN exercise: • **49 out of 56** laboratories passed • **3 out of 56** laboratories did not participate • **4 out of 56** laboratories did not pass *CDC, ONDIEH (NCEH); as of 11/9/09* **25 out of 31** Level 1 and/or Level 2 LRN-C laboratories successfully demonstrated the ability to detect 2 chemical agents in unknown samples during the LRN Emergency Response Pop Proficiency Test (PopPT) Exercise* *Not all Level 1 and Level 2 laboratories are eligible to participate in this exercise. *CDC, ONDIEH (NCEH); as of 8/31/2008* Level 1 LRN-C laboratories took an **average of 98.3 hours** to process and report on 500 samples during the LRN Surge Capacity Exercise (range was 71 to 126 hours) *CDC, ONDIEH (NCEH); 1/9/2009*

Source: Reproduced from U.S. Centers for Disease Control and Prevention. *Public Health Preparedness: Strengthening the Nation's Emergency Response State by State.* Centers for Disease Control and Prevention, Office of Public Health Preparedness and Response. September 2010.

collecting and interpreting data that support detection and response activities, and engaging in preventive actions. The CDC supports state and local entities by providing epidemiologists (26 in fiscal year 2008) and deploying officers from the Epidemic Intelligence Service in Atlanta to assist localities in investigations.[1(p 19)] As with laboratories, however, funds to support epidemiologists have been declining in recent years, and the workforce has suffered. (See **Table 13-2**.)

Communication

A crucial aspect of preparedness is the ability to receive and communicate information rapidly. A state can collect and analyze information with great skill, but if that information is not disseminated in a useful and timely manner, the data themselves lose their purpose. To that end, states have developed methodologies to share public health event data within

TABLE 13-2 Epidemiological Capacity in the 50 States and the District of Columbia Health Departments; 2004–2009

	2004	2009	Percent Decrease
Number of epidemiologists working in state health departments	2,498	2,193	12%
Number of state health departments reporting substantial-to-full capacity in bioterrorism/emergency response	41	37	10%

Source: Reproduced from U.S. Centers for Disease Control and Prevention. *Public Health Preparedness: Strengthening the Nation's Emergency Response State by State.* Centers for Disease Control and Prevention, Office of Public Health Preparedness and Response. September 2010. Available at: http://www.bt.cdc.gov/publications/2010phprep/pdf/complete_PHPREP_report.pdf. Accessed November 14, 2010.

states and developed means to communicate that information to neighboring states and the federal community.

The Health Alert Network (HAN) is a CDC-funded communication system, with partnership from NACCHO and ASTHO, for establishing communications infrastructure to link local and state health departments, first responders, laboratories, and federal entities. HAN is an Internet-based program that enables public health professionals at all levels of government to share disease event data instantaneously, as well as to pass on treatment and response guidelines or warnings regarding urgent health threats.[2] As of 2009, all states had the ability to receive HAN reports, and 96% of state public health departments responded to a HAN test message within 30 minutes (a 23% increase over 2007), demonstrating increased functionality of the system for rapid transmission of crucial information.[1]

States have also increased their capacity over time to communicate disease surveillance information to the federal level using an interoperable electronic system called the National Electronic Disease Surveillance System (NEDSS). The Trust for America's Health reported that in 2004, only 18 states were NEDSS compatible. By 2009, 44 states and Washington, DC, were compatible, while the remaining states were expected to be fully compatible shortly.[3]

Hospital Preparedness

Between 2002 and 2010, the Hospital Preparedness Program at DHHS/ASPR provided approximately $3.6 billion to states to support a series of preparedness priorities.[4,5] States have utilized these funds to improve their ability to handle a rapid rise in medical patients through expanded surge capacity. They have identified alternative care sites for events that may overwhelm existing medical infrastructure, and they have actively registered medical volunteers who could be called on in an emergency.[5] In 2009, 40 states submitted weekly data on the availability of hospital beds for at least 50% of facilities within their states to the National Hospital Available Beds for Emergencies and Disaster (HAvBED) System.[3] Hospitals have planned for supplies, staff, and space in thinking about surge capacity and response to a major public health disaster.

Where state-level hospital preparedness has been weak is in planning for establishing standards of care for emergencies.[5] *Crises standards of care*, as defined by the Institute of Medicine, is the level of medical care provided to patients as justified by specific circumstances as formally declared by a state government for a defined period of time.[6] Crises standards of care brings up difficult challenges around determining how healthcare providers can and should approach mass casualty care in the face of scarce resources; liability concerns;

and unclear protocols for triage, prioritization, and allocation of medical equipment.[3] Only a handful of states have begun the process of planning for and developing these standards.

Community Resilience

By definition, the ability of communities to recover from and be "resilient" in the face of public health emergencies is a local function. The federal government can provide funding and support, but it is up to the local communities to work together and rebound from an event. There is no clear way to measure "resilience." Overall, though, state and local entities have embraced the concept of "seeing the public as a band of hardy survivors and not a panic-stricken mob."[7] How state and local entities have addressed and built stronger social relationships within the communities and worked together to build response and recovery plans has yet to be quantified and no doubt is affected by the ongoing workforce shortages within the public health community.[7]

Response

Local and state officials are the first on the scene to respond to an event. Response in the public health emergency context is about treating populations that are affected by the emergency, containing the event, mitigating the consequences of the event for the rest of the population, and conducting investigations and research to ensure that the authorities will be better prepared in the future. This may be done through support of criminal investigations or through basic scientific research into the origins of a causative agent. Like any other major event, however, it can be assumed that local entities will begin the response, but that as the size or seriousness of the event increases, federal assets will be brought in to assist in, and possibly take control of, the response efforts.

The CDC recently assessed state response capabilities by focusing on performance in exercises and incidents and evaluation and improvement plans. The CDC also focused on the ability of a state to receive and distribute resources from the Strategic National Stockpile. All states had plans to receive items from the Stockpile, and most could activate and rapidly deploy staff to assist in distribution.[1] **Table 13-3** shows the CDC's assessment of state-level response readiness.

CHALLENGES FOR LOCAL AND STATE ENTITIES
Funding

While funding to state and local entities for public health emergency preparedness dramatically increased starting in 2002, it has been decreasing in the past few years. This decrease in funding has translated into specific challenges,

TABLE 13-3 National Snapshot of Response Readiness Activities

Response Readiness: Communication

Communicating emerging health information	**54 out of 54** state and locality public health departments had a 24/7 reporting capacity system that could receive urgent disease reports any time of the day *State and locality data; 10/1/2007–9/30/2008* **48 out of 50** states responded to Health Alert Network (HAN) test message within 30 minutes *CDC, OPHPR (DEO); 7/2009* **47 out of 51** state public health laboratories and DC used HAN or other rapid method (blast email or fax) to communicate with sentinel laboratories and other partners for outbreaks, routine updates, training events, and other applications *APHL; 8/31/2007–8/30/2008* **48%** of approximately 5,500 Epidemic Information Exchange users in 50 states and DC responded to a system-wide notification test within 3 hours *CDC, OPHPR (DEO); 4/3/2008*
Improving public health information exchange	**53 out of 54** states and localities participated in a Public Health Information Network forum (community of practice) to leverage best practices for information exchange *CDC, OSTLTS; as of 9/30/2008*

Response Readiness: Planning

Assessing plans to receive, distribute, and dispense medical assets from the Strategic National Stockpile and other sources	States with acceptable* CDC technical assistance review scores: • **50 out of 50** states for 2008–2009 • **46 out of 50** states for 2007–2008 *A score of 69 or higher (out of 100) indicates state performed in an acceptable range in its plan to receive, distribute, and dispense medical assets. See state fact sheets for individual scores. *CDC, OPHPR (DSNS); 2007–2008 scores are associated with funding from the PHEP cooperative agreement Budget Period 8 (8/13/2007–8/9/2008); 2008–2009 scores are associated with funding from Budget Period 9 (8/10/2008–8/9/2009)* Cities Readiness Initiative (CRI) locations with acceptable* scores: • **18 out of 21** locations in CRI Cohort I (MSAs that enrolled in 2004) • **10 out of 15** locations in CRI Cohort II (MSAs that enrolled in 2005) • **17 out of 36** locations in CRI Cohort III (MSAs that enrolled in 2006) *A score of 69 or higher (out of 100) indicates CRI location performed in an acceptable range in its plan to receive, distribute, and dispense medical assets. See appendix 6 for individual scores. *CDC, OPHPR (DSNS); as of 7/30/2008*
Enhancing response capability for chemical events	**1,941** CHEMPACK nerve-agent antidote containers placed in the 50 states and 4 localities *CDC, OPHPR (DSNS); as of 7/30/2008*
Meeting preparedness standards for local health departments	**150** local health departments in 24 states met voluntary Project Public Health Ready preparedness standards

Response Readiness: Exercises and Incidents

Notifying emergency operations center staff	**53 out of 54** states and localities notified pre-identified staff to fill all eight Incident Command System core functional roles at least twice due to a drill, exercise, or real incident Note: States and localities must report 2 and could report up to 12 notifications. *CDC, OPHPR (DSLR); 8/31/2007–8/9/2008* **53 out of 54** states and localities had pre-identified staff acknowledge notification at least once within the target time of 60 minutes *CDC, OPHPR (DSLR); 8/31/2007–8/9/2008* **52 out of 54** states and localities conducted at least one unannounced notification outside of normal business hours *CDC, OPHPR (DSLR); 8/31/2007–8/9/2008*

TABLE 13-3 National Snapshot of Response Readiness Activities *(Continued)*

Activating the emergency operations center (EOC)	**48 out of 54** states and localities activated their public health emergency operations center (EOC) at least twice as part of a drill, exercise, or real incident Note: States and localities must report 2 and could report up to 12 activations. *CDC, OPHPR (DSLR); 8/31/2007–8/9/2008*
	52 out of 54 states and localities had pre-identified staff report to the public health EOC at least once within the target time of 2.5 hours *CDC, OPHPR (DSLR); 8/31/2007–8/9/2008*
	47 out of 54 states and localities conducted at least one unannounced activation *CDC, OPHPR (DSLR); 8/31/2007–8/9/2008*
Response Readiness: Evaluation	
Assessing response capabilities through after action report/ improvement plans (AAR/IPs)	**52 out of 54** states and localities developed AAR/IPs at least twice following an exercise or real incident Note: States and localities must report 2 and could report up to 12 AAR/IPs. *CDC, OPHPR (DSLR); 8/31/2007–8/9/2008*
	52 out of 54 states and localities developed at least one AAR/IPs within the target time of 60 days *CDC, OPHPR (DSLR); 8/31/2007–8/9/2008*
	51 out of 54 states and localities re-evaluated response capabilities following approval and completion of corrective actions identified in AAR/IPs *CDC, OPHPR (DSLR); 8/31/2007–8/9/2008*

Source: Reproduced from U.S. Centers for Disease Control and Prevention. *Public Health Preparedness: Strengthening the Nation's Emergency Response State by State.* Centers for Disease Control and Prevention, Office of Public Health Preparedness and Response. September 2010. Available at: http://www.bt.cdc.gov/publications/2010phprep/pdf/complete_PHPREP_report.pdf. Accessed November 14, 2010.

primarily in workforce sustainability and laboratory capacity. Researchers at the University of Pittsburg Medical Center (UPMC) have been following federal biodefense funding and found that more than 90% of the biodefense funding budgeted for fiscal year 2011 not only improves biodefense but also improves public health and health care (see **Figure 13-2**).[8] UMPC assesses that since 2001, $61.86 billion has been allocated to biodefense funding. Of the fiscal year 2011 biodefense funding, $4.6 billion is budgeted for DHHS, with the majority allocated to NIH ($1.7 billion) and the second largest amount going to CDC ($1.59 billion).[8] The funding to CDC, which supports the Strategic National Stockpile and the Public Health Emergency Preparedness Cooperative Agreements, has been steadily decreasing over the years. Funding allocated to the Public Health Emergency Preparedness Cooperative Agreement, the mechanism by which CDC funds state and local entities, has declined from a high of $970 million in 2003 to $689 million in 2009.[1]

Workforce

Where the changes in funding hit local and state health departments hardest is in sustaining a workforce adequate for public health preparedness activities. Public health laboratories have had a difficult time sustaining a skilled workforce, with 41% of public health laboratory directors reporting that inability to hire staff was a primary concern.[1] Retaining and paying for skilled epidemiologists at the local and state levels has also been a challenge. CSTE has found that national epidemiologic capacity has dropped significantly in the past 3 years and estimates that approximately 1,500 additional epidemiologists are needed to meet optimal epidemiologic capacity across the country. Eight percent of the highly skilled epidemiologists left state health departments during 2008, and another 17% are anticipated to leave in the next 5 years.[9] In order for state and local public health departments to maintain and grow preparedness services, more attention must be paid to funding streams to support the workforce.

PREPAREDNESS AUTHORITIES

On April 25, 2009, the day that the Director General of the World Health Organization declared H1N1 to be the first public health emergency of international concern under the International Health Regulations, the Office of the Attorney General submitted a memo to President Obama outlining legal

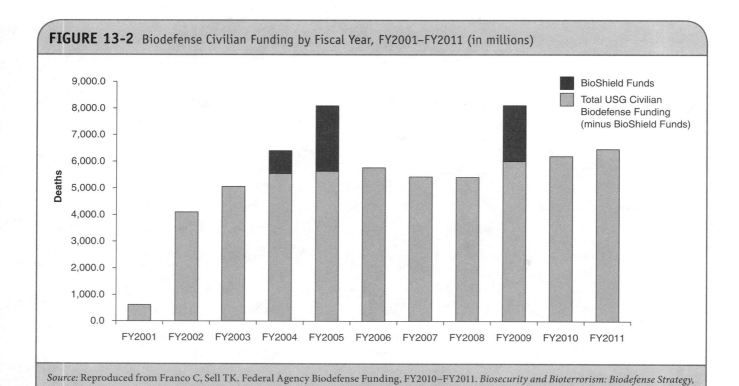

FIGURE 13-2 Biodefense Civilian Funding by Fiscal Year, FY2001–FY2011 (in millions)

Source: Reproduced from Franco C, Sell TK. Federal Agency Biodefense Funding, FY2010–FY2011. *Biosecurity and Bioterrorism: Biodefense Strategy, Practice, and Science.* 2010;8(2):129–149.

authorities for use in response to an outbreak of pandemic influenza. This memo highlighted the different levels of authorities, from federal to local. The Department of Justice memo says that the president and secretary of homeland security can regulate borders by putting restrictions on entry into the country and that DHS and USDA can deny entry of animals into the country. The Federal Aviation Authority and the Transportation Security Administration can close airspace or redirect flights, and the Federal Railroad Administration can impose restrictions on railroads that receive federal funds.[10] The ability to quarantine, however, is a federal, as well as state and local, authority.

QUARANTINE

The ability to quarantine—the separation of people or animals from the rest of the population that are believed to have been exposed to an infectious agent but not yet infected—is a powerful tool in combating and mitigating the effects of an infectious disease outbreak. (See **Box 13-1** for definitions of quarantine and isolation.) The authorities to quarantine lie at both the federal and state levels.

Federal officials can detain, isolate, quarantine, or refuse entry into the United States of individuals reasonably believed to have been infected with an infectious and communicable disease. Most of these authorities pertain to individuals entering the country from abroad. Under Title 42 of the *Code of Federal Regulations*, Parts 70 and 71, the CDC can detail, examine, and release persons coming into the country who may have a communicable disease. To implement this authority, CDC has 20 quarantine stations throughout the country, located at U.S. ports of entry. Large-scale quarantine was last

BOX 13-1 Quarantine and Isolation

Quarantine: Separation and restriction of movement of *well* people or animals that may have been exposed to an infectious agent.

Isolation: Separation and restriction of movement of people or animals that are believed to have a communicable disease.

used during the 1918 pandemic,[11] and the federal quarantine order has only been used a few times in the past 50 years yet was used in the Andrew Speaker case discussed in **Box 13-2**. The president lists the quarantinable diseases in an Executive Order, which currently includes cholera, diphtheria, infectious tuberculosis, plague, smallpox, yellow fever, viral hemorrhagic fevers, SARS, and influenza that is causing or has the potential to cause a pandemic.[12]

Within the country, the authority to quarantine is delegated to the states. Each state has public health laws that allow

---

BOX 13-2 Andrew Speaker Case Study

In 2007, the Andrew Speaker case became headline news, as he evaded public health officials. While the case made for interesting headlines, it also brought up the same concerns as *Jacobson v. Massachusetts*, in that it questioned the extent to which individual liberty needs to be measured against the common good. It also demonstrated that while local public health officials technically have police powers, they are not always comfortable using them. Here are the facts of the case:

In January 2007, Andrew Speaker, 31, was diagnosed with tuberculosis (TB) after receiving chest X-rays for a fall. The X-ray presented an abnormality in his right lung with the appearance of TB, which prompted medical staff to follow through with lab cultures to make an appropriate diagnosis. When Mr. Speaker's lab results came back in March 2007 with a positive reading of TB, Speaker was immediately given standard treatment, and the local health department in Fulton County, Georgia, was notified. By April 25, 2007, Speaker discussed his plans to travel abroad with his physician. On May 10, 2007, only 15 days later, further testing revealed Speaker had multiple-drug-resistant TB (MDR-TB). Following this diagnosis, Speaker was told not to continue with his plans to travel abroad. Against medical advice, Mr. Speaker left for Europe on May 12, 2007, traveling on five different flights to reach his final destination of Italy. During his travel time, the CDC and Fulton County Health Officials attempted to contact him with official travel restrictions but were unsuccessful—they did not realize he had already left the country. On May 17, 2007, previous samples from Speaker were used for more extensive testing while, simultaneously, the CDC was finally informed of his travel to Europe. On May 21 or 22 (time lines fluctuate), results showed he had a further diagnosis of extremely drug-resistant tuberculosis (XDR-TB), and the CDC contacted Customs and Border Protection (CBP) to inform the agency that Speaker was considered a public health risk. A message was then attached to his passport prohibiting his travel on any U.S.-bound flights. Andrew Speaker was contacted May 23, 2007, and told to make his return back to the United States for treatment.

Mr. Speaker was told he could not take a commercial flight back to the United States but could use a private jet. The private jet could cost Speaker up to $100,000—less if he waited for CDC to provide the plane. Speaker was advised to turn himself into Italian authorities until plans could be made. Speaker decided, instead, to make his way back to the United States on his own, taking a circuitous route to try and avoid the expense and authorities.

Clearly marked on a "no-fly list" and having his passport tagged, he was still able to fly into Canada. He rented a car and drove to the border. The U.S. customs official checked his passport and saw the note that he was a public health threat. Mr. Speaker, however, spoke strongly to the customs official and convinced him to let him through because he was not symptomatic. He then drove to New York, where he checked himself into a hospital, was placed under a federal quarantine, and, shortly thereafter, was transferred to National Jewish Hospital, which specialized in TB treatment.

Andrew Speaker caused a public health crisis because he crossed international borders, with the knowledge of his diagnosed MDR-TB (and later XDR-TB) and had the potential of exposing hundreds of people to his infectious disease. This crisis further showed the problems in communication and effectiveness in taking action when there is an infectious outbreak and left room for great improvement in many public health facilities. The case also reopened the debate about individual rights in the face of a public health threat. The actions by Mr. Speaker and the potential threat he was to his many fellow flight passengers left public opinion squarely on the side of public health. Yet Mr. Speaker still claimed that his individual rights were violated; at the same time, the public health community was charged with not acting swiftly or strongly enough.

Sources: Altman LK. Agent at Border, Aware, Let in Man with TB. *The New York Times.* June 1, 2007. Available at: http://www.nytimes.com/2007/06/01/health/01tb.html?_r=3. Accessed November 14, 2010; U.S. House of Representatives, Committee on Homeland Security, Majority Staff. *The 2007 XDR-TB Incident: A Breakdown at the Intersection of Homeland Security and Public Health.* September 2007. Available at: https://www.hsdl.org/?view&doc=82197&coll=limited. Accessed November 14, 2010; and Schwartz J. Tangle of Conflicting Accounts in TB Patient's Odyssey. *The New York Times.* June 2, 2007. Available at: http://www.nytimes.com/2007/06/02/health/02tick.html?scp=4&sq=andrew%20speaker&st=cse. Accessed November 14, 2010.

for quarantine. Local public health departments may also have this authority. Tribes also have police power authorities and can enforce their own isolation and quarantine laws. It is not entirely clear, however, if a state can close its borders to other states and whether the federal government could override such a decision.[10]

Since *Jacobson* was decided in 1905 (see **Box 13-3**), the public health community has been struggling with the proper balance between individual rights and civil liberties and the actions necessary to protect the population. Civil liberties have greatly expanded since quarantine regulations were initially written, and much that is on the books regarding public heath police powers would come as a shock to most of the public. Yet, as public health threats grow, state and local authorities need to have the tools necessary to contain and mitigate the consequences of an emergency. This debate between civil liberties and police powers continues today. In 2005, the Bush administration released revised quarantine regulations for comment. The revised regulations never went into effect, and in 2010, the process was restarted to try once again to find the right balance.

BOX 13-3 *Jacobson v. Massachusetts* (1905): Constitutional Authority to Quarantine

In 1902, Massachusetts passed a law saying all citizens had to either be vaccinated against smallpox or pay a fine. Mr. Jacobson, however, argued that the state could not force him to be vaccinated, and his case ended up in the Supreme Court. The Court decided that by not being vaccinated, Mr. Jacobson was endangering those around him at the same time as receiving the benefits of everyone else being vaccinated. The state was found to have the right to exercise police powers to protect public health.

This holding also applies to the ability of the state to enforce quarantine measures and that individual rights are subject to "restraints and burdens" in order to protect public health.

Source: Jacobson v. Massachusetts, 197 U.S. 11 (1905).

FROM LOCAL TO GLOBAL

All public health is local. Yet diseases know no borders, and a public health emergency in one part of the world may be a public health emergency around the globe in a matter of days. Not only are we interconnected in our threats, but we must then assume that a weakness anywhere in local infrastructure to address public health threats is, in essence, a global weakness.

The approach to public health preparedness to date has relied predominantly on top-down federal policy. These policies have been essential to establishing a culture of preparedness; integrating public health into the national security, homeland security, law enforcement, and emergency response communities; and demonstrating to the global community the importance of the health security interface. Federal entities have engaged the global community in establishing international agreements, communication networks, and funding support mechanisms. And while the local-level public health communities have been engaged in preparedness activities, that level of engagement has varied over time and domestically has not always come with sustainable resources. Internationally, much more investment is still required to appropriately engage local public health entities.

While this book has focused on the role of governments, the key to improving preparedness around the world may lie with the private sector. Government authorities and guidance are essential, but often it is the private sector—with logistical expertise, outreach into the community, and economic and social incentives to assist the populations, particularly during emergencies—that provides real progress. True preparedness will require a whole of nation approach—in the United States and in nations around the world.

Much has been accomplished in public health preparedness over the past decade, and much more still needs to be done. This book has hopefully better prepared the next generation of public health professionals to understand the threats, assess the current activities, and think about how to best prepare for the future.

KEY WORDS

Local and state preparedness
Laboratory capacity
Epidemiologic capacity
Communication
Hospital preparedness
Community resilience
Funding
Workforce
Quarantine

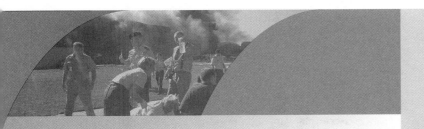

Discussion Questions

1. How do state and local public health professionals contribute to nationwide preparedness? What more (or less) should they be doing?

2. Why are states struggling to maintain epidemiologic capacity?

3. Is the current funding for biodefense at the appropriate level? In a world of limited resources, should more or less be spent?

4. How much power should public health professionals have to quarantine populations? What types of reactions would the population have to being subject to quarantine?

REFERENCES

1. Centers for Disease Control and Prevention, Office of Public Health Preparedness and Response. *Public Health Preparedness: Strengthening the Nation's Emergency Response State by State.* September 2010. Available at: http://www.bt.cdc.gov/publications/2010phprep/pdf/complete_PHPREP_report.pdf. Accessed November 14, 2010.

2. Centers for Disease Control and Prevention, Emergency Preparedness and Response. *The Health Alert Network (HAN).* October 4, 2001. Available at: http://www.bt.cdc.gov/documentsapp/han/han.asp. Accessed November 14, 2010.

3. Trust for America's Health. *Ready or Not? Protecting the Public's Health from Diseases, Disasters, and Bioterrorism.* December 2009. Available at: http://healthyamericans.org/reports/bioterror09/pdf/TFAHReadyorNot 200906.pdf. Accessed November 14, 2010.

4. U.S. Department of Health and Human Services, Office of the Assistant Secretary for Preparedness and Response. *HHS Fact Sheet: FY10 Hospital Preparedness Program (HPP).* September 20, 2010. Available at: http://www.phe.gov/Preparedness/planning/hpp/Pages/fy10hpp.aspx. Accessed November 14, 2010.

5. *U.S. Government Accountability Office. Emergency Preparedness: State Efforts to Plan for Medical Surge Could Benefit from Shared Guidance for Allocating Scarce Medical Resources.* January 25, 2010. Available at: http://www.gao.gov/new.items/d10381t.pdf. Accessed November 14, 2010.

6. Institute of Medicine (IOM). *Guidance for Establishing Crisis Standards of Care for Use in Disaster Situations.* Washington, DC: National Academies Press, 2009. Available at http://books.nap.edu/openbook.php?record_id=12749&page=R1.

7. Schoch-Spana M. Community Resilience for Catastrophic Health Events. *Biosecurity and Bioterrorism: Biodefense Strategy, Practice, and Science.* 2008;6(2):129–130.

8. Franco C, Sell TK. Federal Agency Biodefense Funding, FY2010–FY2011. *Biosecurity and Bioterrorism: Biodefense Strategy, Practice, and Science.* 2010;8(2):129–149.

9. Council of State and Territorial Epidemiologists. *2009 National Assessment of Epidemiology Capacity: Findings and Recommendations.* Available at: http://www.cste.org/dnn/LinkClick.aspx?fileticket=%2BS%2FEifgcbmM% 3D&tabid=36&mid=1496. Accessed November 14, 2010.

10. U.S. Department of Justice, Office of the Attorney General. *Memorandum of Legal Authorities for Use in Response to an Outbreak of Pandemic Influenza.* National Conference of State Legislatures. April 25, 2009. Available at: http://www.ncsl.org/Portals/1/Documents/health/attorneygeneral_flu.pdf. Accessed November 14, 2010.

11. Centers for Disease Control and Prevention. *Legal Authorities for Isolation and Quarantine.* January 29, 2010. Available at: http://www.cdc.gov/quarantine/AboutLawsRegulationsQuarantineIsolation.html. Accessed November 14, 2010.

12. Centers for Disease Control and Prevention. *Questions and Answers on the Executive Order Adding Potentially Pandemic Influenza Viruses to the List of Quarantinable Diseases.* February 3, 2010. Available at: http://www.cdc.gov/quarantine/qa-executive-order-pandemic-list-quarantinable-diseases.html. Accessed November 14, 2010.

Glossary

Agroterrorism: the threat or use of biological or chemical agents against the agricultural industry or food supply system.

Australia Group: informal group of countries that creates a list of common export controls for chemical and biological agents and related equipment to harmonize national export control measures.

Biodefense: measures taken to prevent, detect, respond to, and recover from harm caused by a biological agent.

Biorisk: the chance that any type of adverse event involving a biological agent leading to potential harm will occur.

Biosafety: process of maintaining safe conditions to prevent people and the environment from being exposed to hazardous biological agents.

Biosafety Level: practices, equipment, and infrastructure associated with safely containing biohazardous materials or agents; levels correspond to actions that must be taken to contain increasingly dangerous agents.

Biosecurity: process to reduce or eliminate the ability of a biological agent to adversely affect human, animal, or plant health; the protection and control of agents to prevent against loss, theft, misuse, or intentional release.

Biological Agent: any microorganism, including bacteria, viruses, fungi, rickettsia and Chlamydia, prions, and protozoa, that are capable of causing harm, death, or some disease in a living organism.

Biological Warfare: military use of a biological agent by a state to cause death or harm to humans, animals, or plants.

Biological Weapons Convention: international treaty prohibiting the development, production, proliferation, and retention of biological or toxin weapons.

Biosurveillance: any method to detect and monitor a biological incident, disease activity or threat to health, whether of intentional or natural origin.

Bioterrorism: the threat or use of a biological agent typically by a non-state actor to cause death or harm to humans, animals, or plants, specifically targeting civilian populations or resources.

Blister Agent: type of chemical weapon causing irritation of the skin and mucous membrane.

Blood Agent: type of chemical weapon causing seizures and respiratory and cardiac failure in high doses.

Category A, B, and C Threat Agents: categories assigned to the major known biological threat agents, based on the amount of morbidity and mortality the agents are capable of causing, ease of weaponization, previous history of weaponization, and need for specific response planning.

Chemical Weapons Convention: international treaty banning the use, proliferation, and stockpiling of chemical weapons.

Chemical Warfare: use of chemical substance to intentionally harm or kill humans, plants, or animals.

Choking Agent: type of chemical weapon causing damage to the lungs, including pulmonary edema and hemorrhage.

Code of Conduct: guidelines that organizations and individuals voluntarily agree to abide by, that set standards for behavior.

Communicable disease: a disease transmitted from person to person.

Cooperative Threat Reduction: efforts conducted primarily through the Departments of Defense and State to engage countries to reduce threats, particularly around weapons of mass destruction, biosecurity, and biosurveillance.

Decontamination: the process of eliminating an infectious or toxic agent that may constitute a public health risk from either a living or inanimate surface.

Disease: illness or medical condition that presents harm to a living being.

Disease Outbreak: an occurrence of disease greater than would otherwise be expected at a particular time and place.

Dual Use: research, agents, technologies, equipment, or information that can be used for both legitimate scientific purposes or for malevolent use.

Emerging Infectious Disease: an infectious disease that newly appears in a population or that has been known for some time, but rapidly increasing in incidence or geographic range.

Epidemiology: the study of patterns of health and illness and associated factors at the population level.

Epidemic: (see Disease Outbreak)

Executive Order: a presidential directive with the authority of a law that directs and governs actions by executive officials and agencies.

Federal Emergency Management Agency: the U.S. federal agency responsible for responding to national emergencies, including natural disasters.

Geneva Protocol: international treaty that bans the use of chemical and biological agents in war.

Healthcare Worker: someone whose job involves close contact with patients or patient items. These include a variety of professions, such as clinicians, therapists, social workers, pharmacists, and other technicians.

Health Security: per the World Health Organization, health security is the activities and intersect of disciplines necessary to minimize the impact of acute public health events on populations, economies, and political stability.

Health Status: all aspects of physical and mental health and their manifestations in daily living, including impairment, disability, and handicap.

Health Threat: an environmental, biological, chemical, radiological, or physical risk to public health in the context of national or global security.

Homeland Defense: the protection of U.S. territory, populations, and infrastructure against external threats or aggression.

Homeland Security: the actions and policies associated with preventing, deterring, responding to, and recovering from aggressions targeted at U.S. territory, populations, and infrastructure.

Homeland Security Presidential Directive: a directive from the George W. Bush Administration's Homeland Security Council that recorded or communicated presidential decisions and policies related to homeland security.

Incidence: number of new cases of illness or disease during a specific period of time in a specific population.

International Atomic Energy Agency: an international organization, reporting to the United Nations General Assembly and Security Council that promotes the peaceful and safe use of nuclear energy, while inhibiting the intentional, offensive use of nuclear weapons.

International Health Regulations (2005): an international treaty obligating all Member States of the World Health Organization to detect, report, and respond to potential public health emergencies of international concern, and improve global health security through international collaboration and communication to detect and contain public health emergencies at the source.

Intelligence Community: the collection of 16 agencies, offices, programs, and bureaus that collect, analyze, and report on intelligence information in support of policy makers across the government.

Isolation: separation and restriction of movement of people or animals that are believed to have a communicable disease.

Medical Countermeasures: pharmaceutical products and equipment, such as drugs, vaccines, and ventilators to both prevent the harmful effects of a biological, chemical, or radiological agent, and mitigate the consequences for those who become ill.

Medical Intelligence: collection, analysis, and reporting of health threats and issues, including infectious disease threats, environmental health risks, data to support force health protection, and the medical information on individuals with regional and international importance.

National Security: the actions and policies associated with safeguarding the territorial integrity, existence, and safety of the State.

National Security Council Directives: types of executive orders (with varying names depending on the administration) done with the advice and consent of the National Security Council that have the effect of law.

Nerve Agent: a type of chemical weapon that primarily acts on the nervous system, causing seizures and death.

National Incident Management System: a document providing for standardized incident management protocols for responding to any type of emergency at all levels of government.

National Response Framework: a broad national plan for preparedness and response to disasters and emergencies.

Notifiable Disease: a disease that must be reported to a public health authority, either by statute or regulation.

Nuclear Nonproliferation Treaty: an international treaty to limit the spread of nuclear weapons, encourage disarmament, and foster the right to peacefully use nuclear technology.

Nuclear Weapon: an explosive device powered by a nuclear reaction.

Pandemic: an infectious disease that spreads through human populations across a large region, over multiple continents.

Personal Protective Equipment: clothing and equipment that create a barrier between humans and health hazards, such as surgical masks.

Population health: health outcomes of a group of individuals, including the distribution of such outcomes within a group.

Preparedness: the actions and policies associated with preventing, protecting against, responding to, and recovering from a major event.

Prevalence: total number of cases of a disease or illness in the population at a given time.

Public Health Emergency: an acute event capable of causing large scale morbidity and mortality, either immediately or over time. These events have the ability to overwhelm normal public health capabilities.

Public Health Emergency of International Concern: a technical term associated with the International Health Regulations (2005), determined through an algorithm and defined as an event that constitutes a public health risk to other nations and potentially requires an internationally coordinated response.

Public Health Preparedness: the actions and policies associated with preventing, protecting against, responding to, and recovering from public health emergencies.

Quarantine: separation and restriction of movement of well people or animals that may have been exposed to an infectious agent.

Radiological Event: an explosion or other release of radioactivity.

Select Agent: List of biological agents, subject to federal regulations, that may pose a severe threat to public health and security.

Stafford Act: the principal document for U.S. federal authority for assisting states and local governments in responding to any type of disaster.

Strategic National Stockpile: federal stockpile of drugs, vaccines, and medical equipment that can be rapidly deployed to any locality in the country in response to a public health emergency.

Surge Capacity: ability of clinical care facilities and laboratories to accommodate a sharp increase in patients and samples during a public health emergency.

Synthetic Biology: the design and creation of biological components and systems that do not naturally exist.

Toxin: poisonous substances produced by living entities.

United Nations Security Council Resolution 1540: resolution obligating United Nations Member States to ensure they do not support non-state actors in their efforts to develop, acquire, possess, or use nuclear, chemical, or biological weapons.

Weapons of Mass Destruction: weapons that cause large scale destruction, generally including nuclear, radiological, chemical, and biological weapons. May also include high yield explosives.

World Health Organization: the directing and coordinating authority for health within the United Nations system. It is responsible for providing leadership on global health matters, shaping the health research agenda, setting norms, articulating evidence-based policy options, and providing technical support to countries.

Zoonosis: any disease that is transmitted from animal to human.

Index

List of Figures

List of Boxes

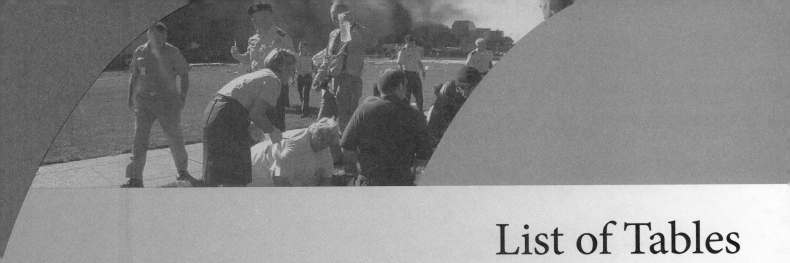

List of Tables